Makeup Artist Manual: From Beginner to Pro

Nina Mua

MAKE UP

Table of Contents

Table of Contents 2

CHAPTER 1:
Shading and The Undertone 3

CHAPTER 2:
Corrective Make-up 13

CHAPTER 3:
Eyebrows 43

CHAPTER 4:
Eye-Shadow 56

CHAPTER 5:
Cheeks 78

CHAPTER 6:
Lips 91

CHAPTER 7:
Putting it all together 117

CHAPTER 8:
Mature Make-Up 127

CHAPTER 9:
Bridal Make-up 140

CHAPTER 10:
Airbrush 144

CHAPTER 1:
Shading and The Undertone

All of the shades that make-up bases come in, are subtlety. They come in a large variety, just as the human skin. A make-up artist needs an understanding of the different variations that can come from the many bases in make-up and that is why this lesson has been created.

This is also intended to teach the make-up artists how to use the information provided in conducting the base tone and skin match. The two elements that are necessary, and most visualized for accuracy in a base tone and skin match are the undertone and shading.

The darkness and lightness in a base is the shade. You can observe a gray scale, and visualize the difference in the shades. At the beginning of the gray scale notice how it starts with 10% and increases by 10 with each of the following increments until it reaches 100%. Making it obvious that white would be at the 0% increment, while black is the 100% increment.

Every shade possible to cover the shade of human faces and all base shades will be located somewhere on the gray

MAKE UP

scale. A gray scale merely represents the base shades from the lighter to the darker shades, and is not itself a color.

Gray Scale

Take notice in the following gray scale how each increment is 10% more in darkness as the previous one. Zero percent equaling the shade of white, and 100% equaling the shade of black.

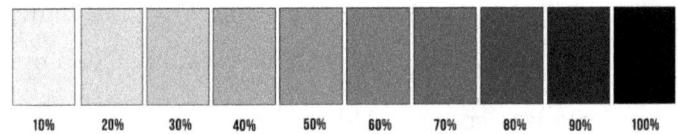

Exercise For Shades

Taking a series of cream products and placing them in order from left to right, starting with the lightest shade first and ending with the darkest. You will be able to see the subtle and obvious difference in each shade.

Align the bases so that they can be identified, and though there may be times that seem a little confusing, you will be able to use the gray scale to figure it out. After correctly having them in order, record your results on the gray scale worksheet.

Next, you are going to use the worksheet out of the workbook provided. You are to take a small dab from each

MAKE UP

of the containers using the palette tool (knife) placing it in the area designated for that base color. You will do this with all of the bases, in order from left (lightest) to right (darkest).

You will find labels for each base, fill them in, giving the assigned number or name for each. As you progress everything will become more apparent.

NOTE:

Remember to wipe the palette blade after placing each base, and before moving to the next one. This is important in order to keep from getting the bases mixed in with another one.

Undertone

In order to match skin tone perfectly, you will also go by an element referred to as the undertone. The undertone is what is used in getting the intrinsic color match of the skin. You're going to find that, while most skin tones are easily detected, there are others that will not be so easy to determine. Many skin tones will have a rich undertone, but not all.

Colors of the undertone are going to represent them self in a variety of shades ranging anywhere from a light pinkish to a dark reddish color, and as the shade appears higher up on the darker scale the undertones can range anywhere from yellowish to a greenish (and can sometimes appear in a blueish form). As you can see, undertones can be produced in a great variety of different colors. However, you're going to find a majority of undertones are going to be in the olive color.

Colors of the undertones can be different in one series than it is in another series, as with one line of product to another product line. There may be some lines of product and series that have more undertones than others. That is why aligning them in order left to right, and comparing on the gray scale by increments is going to help distinguish the ones that are not so easy to notice.

Good lighting is absolutely necessary to effectively see the subtleness that can occur in each of the base shades. Always have a well lit area to work in. Sometimes it may even be necessary to place your undertone on a sheet of white paper and slowly move from side to side. By distinguishing a background that is neutral, it will help in determining the difference in the undertones as well.

It's suggested to use a white cloth to cover the model while applying the make-up. Having a white back ground will show the skin of the model much better, and will prove beneficial when matching skin tone and undertones.

MAKE UP

Exercise:

Using a series of cream products, align the bases in order, left to right, starting with the yellowish to greenish, with the least yellow being on the left, and ending up with the darker of the green on the right.

Once the bases are identified, use the yellowish to green worksheet, writing your results on the worksheet, recording them as usual.

Now, remove a dab of base out of the bottle with the palette tool, putting it in the designated spot found on your worksheet, in order from left to right.

After doing this you will notice that the difference in the undertones are more noticeable. Now you are going to finish the rest of the spots on the scale by increments of 10, completing the entire scale. Don't forget to put down the number and/or name of the base for each in the correct spot provided. Being sure to wipe the palette in between each of the bases.

Note:

The shade will not matter in this exercise, we are only working with the undertones at this time.

As you move along in this lesson, keep in mind that the

shade is not the same thing as the undertone.

When aligning the undertones you may find that the order can be very different then they were in placing the shades.

Matching Skin Tone

In this lesson you will learn the importance of knowing and developing an eye for matching the base and skin tone. This is the first step in this lesson, and should be well learned before going any further. You will need to observe the skin shade in an overall matter when it comes to people.

This includes noticing if the neck, arms, and legs are lighter than the face area, or maybe they are darker than those areas. Also, you will at times run into a predicament where the face itself may not be all the same color (this could be due to a defect at birth or scaring from an accident).

There can be a big difference in one's facial color. Now, you have to learn where you would put this on a gray scale. This will be done by paying great attention to the colors in the undertones.

Ask yourself, how much pinkish is there? And, how much reddish color is there? Then, how much greenish is there?

In order to match the skin tone it will consist of using a combination of the shades and the undertones. Keep in mind that most of the world's population will have to some extent a little greenish (olive tent) undertone to their skin. Don't let yourself get distracted by the different variety of shades you may find in faces. The main question here would be, which one of the shades should be used to match the base?

In the initial examination of one's skin you may find that the skin has a redness, this could be caused by various reasons, such as: irritation, blemishes, blood vessels, veins that are closer to skin than usual, and even blueness showing around eyes. It is important not to let these distractions take away your ability to find the real undertone color of their skin.

Sometimes you will find a face that has a little bit of difference in the undertone and shade more in one area, than in another. Especially, in the crossover area (the area where the face and neck come together). More so if someone wears their base with a sunscreen, this sort of thing can be very noticeable during summer months. But, having a base that matches up properly to begin with, is going to reduce, and possibly even eliminate the issue.

You are going to find that most people's skin match is

MAKE UP

best done in the area in front of the ear, and towards the bottom of the ear. This is where the undertone will prove to be at its clearest. Since this is the area where the face and neck join, it is going to let the make-up artists get a full view of the shade and undertone in a picture as a whole.

Exercise:

You will need to understand the difference in matching the different bases, and the combinations of bases, which there are to match, as well as how it will relate to the undertone and shading. Take a look at the forearm, now look at the underarm. Notice how there is a slight change in the darkness of one side and the other side being lighter in color? Usually, the forearm will be darkest in color.

You will be able to observe the differences when in a well lit area. Most people will have some differences, mostly due to over exposure from constant sunlight. The amount of difference of course, will depend on the amount of exposure they have had.

Start out by picking a cream base that matches closest in undertone and shade to the outer arm (forearm). If you decide that you haven't came up with a match, then you will begin combining or mixing in order to get a proper match.

MAKE UP

Shade

What if the base is too dark or too light on the skin? Too light - You will need to add just a dab of a base that is darker, and mix it well, you can use the palette tool for this part. Then, simply add to it, a little at a time until you reach the desired shade. If it is too dark- You will do the same thing only using a lighter base, not forgetting to mix well.

Undertone

If you can't find a perfect match for the base, you will then have to proceed to using combinations, and mixing to locate the proper color. Remember, this is done by using the two bases that are closest in match. If you have one base that is slightly lighter, and another that is slightly darker, try mixing these two together.

It is important that the artist come up with the correct base colors. Always use the palette tool when mixing colors, and don't forget to wipe the palette when changing to a single color, or changing colors in general.

Using one of the make-up sponges, apply a dab of base on the outer side of the forearm. You will keep taking a base, and mixing with the previous base until you achieve a perfect match. You can tell when you have reached a perfect match, because the shade and base color will no

MAKE UP

longer appear, it blends in so well that it has actually disappeared.

This is the objective, for the base to no longer be noticeable, and for it to have a natural appearance. When this has been accomplished it is time to do the same thing on the underarm(or inside the forearm).

CHAPTER 2:
Corrective Make-up

There is an advanced technique used in the process of corrective utilization with different methods when it comes to highlights, shadows, and corrective colors (meaning concealers), to fix the negative aspects of the ones that have an offset appearance on the face.

It is a necessity to learn the application process of the bases, for that is the beginning of being able to develop a make-up of beauty.

Once you are aware of the initial start of it all, you can then begin with the techniques to do any correcting that is necessary.

The appearance of the facial area can be improved upon in great detail if you have the knowledge of basic base procedures and the technique of correctness.

Once this chapter has been completed by the make-up artists, it is going to give them the ability to conceal, correct, and use the means of camouflaging for any aspects of negativeness in the facial area.

MAKE UP

Sculptural Light

The first step would be in studying the lighting principles, and chiaroscuro (shade) theory, and to be observant to the things around us. Next, to use the techniques learned here in actual make-up applications.

The main key in using techniques for corrective make-up has everything to do with the shade and lighting, and the understanding of it. A make-up artist should be able to manipulate shade and light well enough to give off the illusion of objects, such as three dimensional ones.

And the artist must in the same way be able to manipulate shade and light in order to correct any negative spots that have excess highlights or shadows within the facial area.

Depending on the lighting, what we see when looking at a face comes from the reflection that that lighting puts off. And due to each face having different shapes, that lighting is going to reflect off the faces showing a entirely different pattern.

MAKE UP

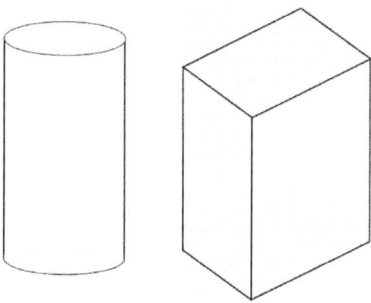

When an artist is painting a portrait they are able to change the position of the lighting used, and they manipulate that lighting to their benefit.

Positioning the lighting to prevail certain shadows and highlights where ever the artist wants to put them in the portrait. The artist thus, uses the lighting to position the shadows and highlights within the portrait.

Without the use of a light source in shadowing and highlighting, a portrait would not look real, it would be bland in appearance. The difference in an artist that paints a portrait, and an artist of make-up is that make-up artists doesn't usually have the opportunity to position the shading and lighting in the places they need it the most.

Make-up artists will have the option of placing their light source, generally, either in front of the object or above, leaving their options to be very limited. Knowing where to put the shadows and highlights will depend once again on where the light itself is. Once this is established however, they can surmise where to place the shades and highlights on the face.

The Two Dimensional World

The make-up artist must have the knowledge in the differences of a two dimensional, and a three dimensional world in the television and film industries. Have you ever noticed that when you see yourself in a mirror you are only seeing point blank, the part that is facing the mirror? Notice how it seems to be so lifeless, or without any type of shape? You are not able to see the different angles (not without more mirrors). That's because you are seeing yourself at an angle of 180 degree. In other words, in a two dimensional angle.

Next, while closing one of your eyes you are going to take your finger and place it before your face, slowly move the finger from one side to another, switching up as you go.

Without the use of both eyes you do not have the ability to accurately describe the depth, or rather to precept the depth. Being able to see the in-depth of something gives us the ability to see around it so to speak. Actually, it's like having the capability to observe half of an object at a time. What we can then see are the dimensions of depth, width,

MAKE UP

and height.

A camera of three dimensions is really merely two cameras that have been put together using the same distance apart as is between the eyes, and each side is recording in a different color.

If we put something in front of the cameras, one side of the camera will be shooting it from the same view as we would be seeing it from our left eye. And, of course, the other side of the camera is shooting it the same as our right eye is seeing it.

There are specially made glasses to wear when looking at things in a three dimensional perspective, like going to see a movie that's in 3D. Without wearing the glasses to see the movie you cannot grasp all the objects you are meant too. A camera shoots a picture through one lens, and it is projected through to a flat screen.

This means, as a make-up artist, you will be able to make the audience believe what they are seeing is only painted on a face, instead of it really being there. This is because the audience sees an illusion of depth that the make-up artist has created. The audience can't see the depth itself, for they do not possess this ability.

MAKE UP

Curved and Flat Surfaces

Let's take a look at the following two objects: a cylinder, and a box.

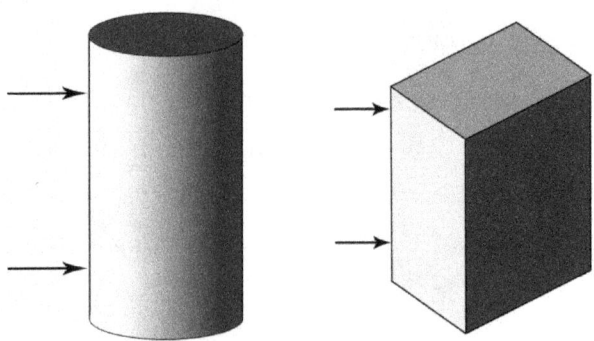

Although the two objects have an out-line which gives a clue to their shapes, it is the highlights and shadows that are reflecting the box and cylinder making it possible in determining the two objects true shape.

The effect that makes it possible for a viewer to see the objects comes from the illumination of a light source, in the directions the arrows are going. When the light is upon the object it makes it reflect back to the viewers eyes.

Being able to see the object is only possible because the light that is provided allows it. Observing this in absolute darkness would not let you see anything. Pay close attention to how the light falls on the subject, notice that it isn't falling evenly onto them.

MAKE UP

The areas in darkness are in an area that is not getting light. Those that are fully noticeable have the light directly on them. As the curves of the surface slowly moves away from the source of light, the shadow gradually increases around the cylinder. You are going to see the same in the gray scale as far as transition is concerned.

Making it possible for the viewer to know the direction that the light may be coming from. Regardless if the surface is curved, irregular, or flat. The shape of the object is now revealed.

If you pay close attention to the box and the cylinder in the following illustration, you will see that the objects are highlighted, and in a shadow. However, the shadow and the highlights reflect in a different way on the box, as well as the cylinder.

Indicating the surface of the cylinder is curved is the way the light shifts gradually moving from the light into the shadow. You can notice the sudden shift from light to dark on the box, indicating a flat hard surface, sharp edges, and also sharp corners.

Known as the hard edge, it is the sharp part that falls between the shadow, and the highlighting. The soft edge, is known by the gradual shifting, that falls between the shadow, and the highlighting.

The two patterns of these shadows and highlights point

MAKE UP

directly to the make-up that has been corrected.

Example:

Shadow Cylinder Pattern

Observe the pattern of the shadow around the cylinder. The area that is lightest on the cylinder is indicated by the W. Showing that this area is the part which receives the most amount of light.

The area that receives the lesser amount of light is indicated by the X. Whereas the slightly darker area is represented by the Y. Last, is the darkest area, meaning it receives no light at all, it is represented by the Z

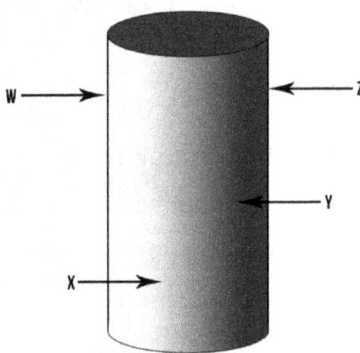

You should be noticing by now that the light source becomes lesser as the surface curves move away from the light. Noticing, that the shadow that is deepest, is opposite of the source of the light.

MAKE UP

Example:

Nasolabial Fold

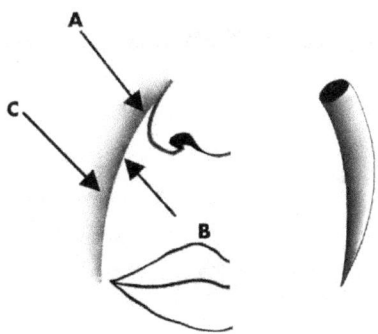

The largest wrinkle pattern on the face is in general, the nasolabial fold. It extends from the corner of the lips up to the outer part of the nostril, as seen in the illustration above. In the illustration above the nasolabial is well developed and creates a crease/fold around the general area of the skin.

Notice how the fold has been created with a shadow of a hard edge (arrow A) and next to it a hard edge using highlights (arrow B).The fold on the outside fades gradually (arrow C).

You will find this shadow and highlighting pattern is

MAKE UP

like the shadow and highlighting pattern that's in the cylinder illustration. The transition is gradual in the crease of the hard edge to the softer edge around the outside by the wrinkle.

Example:

Shadow pattern "Soft Edge to Soft Edge"

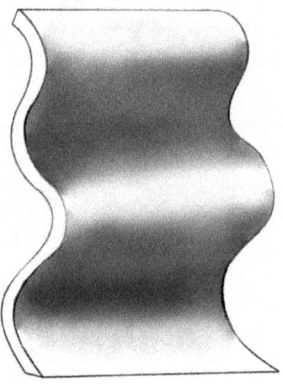

In the shadow "soft edge to soft edge" pattern there is no wrinkles due to there not being a hard edge. You can see that the lighting falls unevenly over the object.

If the area of the surface does not get any light, then they are considered to be in a shadow. Otherwise, it would be considered to be fully visible, should the light fall directly over the shadow.

MAKE UP

There is gradual shadow increase in this object, where the surface is curving away from the light. This shows that the transition is gradual to the shadow from the light. You can find this on the gray scale.

Example:

Soft edge to soft edge- Labeled

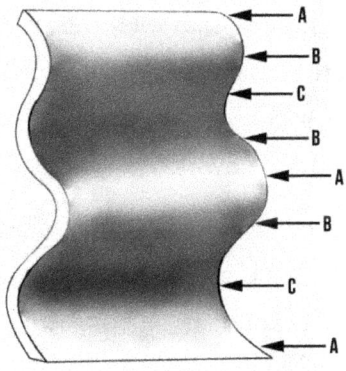

You're at positive A, this is where the highlight will begin, and slowly becomes darker to reach positive B. Now at positive C, the shadow has reached the darkest.

For the soft edge to soft edge effect the highlights, and shadows will gradually be shifting, to shadows from the highlights.

MAKE UP

Shadows and Highlights

Example:

Front View - Face With Shadow

You are going to find that no one's head, and no one's face is going to be exact. This is why the shadows and highlighted patterns in the following is going to vary from one another.

For this shadow example, the pattern will apply directly with corrective make-up. Look at the cheek-bone; it has highlights at the top, and the cheek-bone has some shadowing just below it.

Take notice that the shadows and highlights are soft edges. Doesn't the cheek-bone remind you of the cylinder? Without the hard edges, of course.

Shadows and highlight patterns reflect off the forehead, and have soft edges. An uneven effect is given to the forehead in this pattern. Keep in mind that the pattern for shadow, and the forehead is going to be different with everyone.

The high and low areas of the forehead can be felt by rubbing the finger across it. With the higher areas reflecting more light, and the lower areas reflecting less light. The lower areas tend to have a shadow, due to not

MAKE UP

having a lot of light.

So, they reflect less light as well, which tends to give the forehead an uneven appearance, the same with other areas of the face. These areas become more announce as one ages.

There are a variety of products , along with many application techniques that can help in creating shadows and highlights.

Cream Application

You can use cream products to add the shadows, and highlights once the base has been applied.

Highlights:

Using lighter shades of the base with the undertone series can be used to highlight a position, unless you have another product that has been made especially for highlighting, if so, you may use it.

Usually, this type of product will have a little bit of a tint, possibly orange or yellow. You will use a palette tool for mixing the base and highlights together, blending well.

Once again, don't forget to wipe your palette clean before going to another color, to keep from contaminating the other colors. Go with a shade that is lighter than the

MAKE UP

base and take a small dab to mix with the base chosen, this should give you a relationship of a base tone.

You may also use any of these products alone. Use just a dab at a time carefully putting over what base is already on with a sponge.

Shadows:

To have the shadow colors work their best try and remember to use a dab of gray in your shading colors. If using shades that are dark for the base, and they are from a series of undertones that are the same, you can use them for your shadowing positions.

When using colors for shadowing always blend into the base. Using a dab of shadow color mixed with the base can help you to achieve the base tone relationship.

Setting The Base:

After using the base, and using the cream product, it's time to powder it up! Using powder is necessary in order to set the make-up. Using a loose powder, light in color will work nicely. It isn't going to change the color of cream product that was previously applied.

MAKE UP

Powder Application

Loose powder is used to set the make-up, and should be applied after the base, letting it set completely. This has to be done before the shadows and/or highlights. You will be providing a consistent surface for the powder, as powder has a tendency to slide right over other powder, thus, making it ready for a powder application, or product.

Highlights:

You can find powdered shadow and powdered highlights if you look hard enough. There are companies that make these products, but, if they're not available to you, you can use a lighter shade of shadow, or even some colors can be used for highlights.

Always build your applications by using small increments, use a little, blend, and use a little more and blend, and etc., giving the make-up artist control of the process.

Remember, it will be easier to add a little should the need arise, rather than go to the trouble of removing anything, should there be to much.

Shadows:

Eye shadow that is darker in shade, and containing a

little gray will work just fine. And, as always, build up your application in little increments at a time.

Example:

Negative Hard Edge/Soft Edge

It is the job of the make-up artist to balance out any uneven areas on the face. You will do this using shadows and highlights, they can be used to counteract any previous shadows and highlights that had a negative effect. Like an unwanted raise in the forehead. Or you might have an unwanted depression.

If you should have a shadow pattern that is negative and needs to be corrected it will be necessary to get a lighter color than the base color. This is going to give off more light, remember, the face shadow already reflects lesser light than most other areas of the face.

If you come across a shadow that needs to be eliminated or reduced you can apply highlighting color on that area, it will change the effect of that shadow. There needs to be a base tone relation. If the base tone and the highlight have the same or near the same undertone then there is a relationship.

To find out what can be used as a highlight for a particular base, check the base worksheets found in the chapter on base.

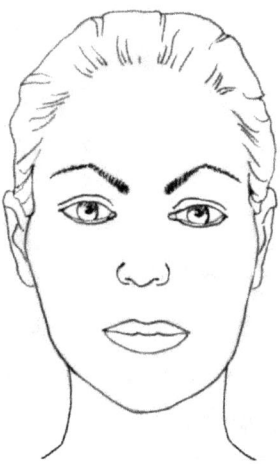

The Nasolabial Fold Correction

The nasolabial fold has a soft and a hard edge. If it is used, the highlight is to be put on the shadow. Placing a hard edge of the highlight into the hard edge of the shadow (arrow A). The highlight will start to fade as soon as the shadow does (arrow B),

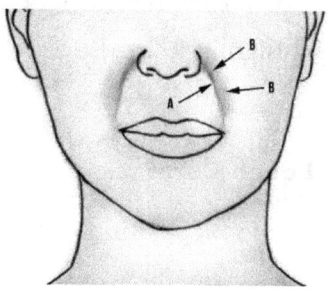

Be careful that the highlights hard edge doesn't go

MAKE UP

further out, or become more noticeable than the shadows hard edge. Should this happen, then the work already done to correct any defaults will be canceled out. In other words, the effect of the highlight will no longer apply.

Application:

The highlight color can be applied with the use of a make-up brush (shadow brush), you can also use a concealers brush. In this case, you will want to put a dab of the product on the palette tool, and get the highlight on the brush by stroking it across the palette tool. Distribute evenly on both sides of the brush.

Positioning the brush at the very top of the hard edge (by the nasolabial fold), and pulling the brush in a downward motion, right on the hard edge all the way to the bottom of the shadow. Gently blend the highlight with the shadow blending until the highlight is blended in so well that it makes the shadow fade away. Always keep the hard edge of a highlight hard.

The Eye Pouch Correction

There is a shadow position called the eye pouch. This is another one of those flaws you may come across when putting on someone's face. You can correct this by doing

MAKE UP

the same thing you did to correct the nasolabial fold.

Look at (arrow A), now using the hard edge take the highlight and place on the hard edge of the shadow, and blend together working towards the eye (arrow B).

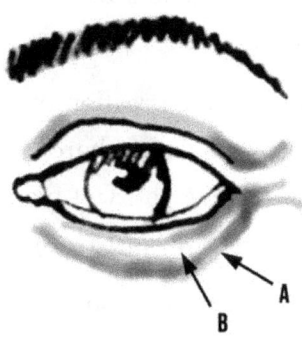

MAKE UP

Upper Lid Correction

On the outside, and in the upper corner find the eyelid, notice that it has developed a shadow pattern. This pattern has given the effect that makes the eye appear to be drooping. That appearance becomes more obvious when the hard edge develops.

Begin doing the correction of the drooping effect. Begin by putting the highlights hard edge on the shadows hard edge (arrow A). Now you will blend them together working towards that eye-brow (arrow B).

Remember, anytime you have a negative pattern of a shadow and its hard edge, you will be able to correct it exactly the way you have been learning in this lesson.

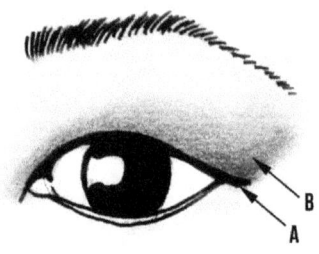

MAKE UP

Eye Ledge Correction

When the area under the eye gets recessed (it could also be just behind the lower part of the orbital rim), it can cause a shadow position. Which causes a hard edge on the shadow at the point where the tissue and the orbital rim meet, right below the eye. It is here that the shadow will begin to disappear, fading downward and backing off of the eye.

You will simply use the same correction pattern used in all of the soft edge/hard edge shadowing. You will start by putting the highlight (arrow A) hard edge onto the shadow's hard edge and begin blending together working downward, backing away from the eye (arrow B).

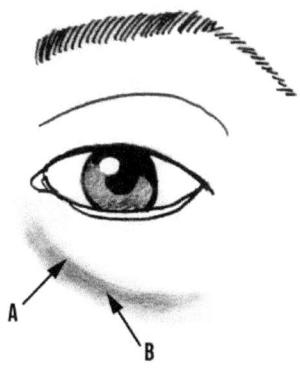

MAKE UP

Correction Of The Jaw-Line

You can define the jaw-line by using a combination of highlight and shadow, as well as the nose and cheek-bone areas.

Application:

Take a look at (arrow A) notice how the use of highlight on the shadow area seems to correct it?

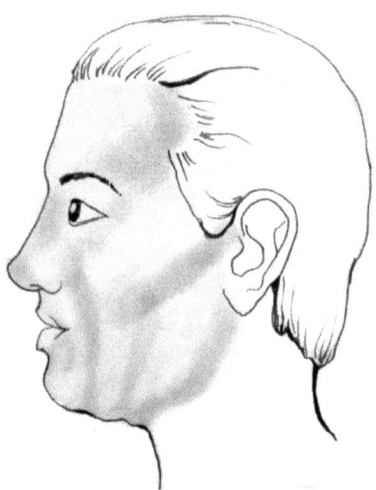

Now look at (arrow B) it shows you what you can do in cases where the highlight alone in the shadow areas appears not to be working for you, and suggests that it could be necessary to use some shadow. If this is the case, take a little shadow, an add a soft edge. This can

MAKE UP

sometimes correct the problem. Blend it in well, until there are no shadows left with a hard edge.

Cheek-Bone Corrections

Shadows and highlights can be used to accentuate the cheek bones. Take a look at the following illustration of the cheek bone area:

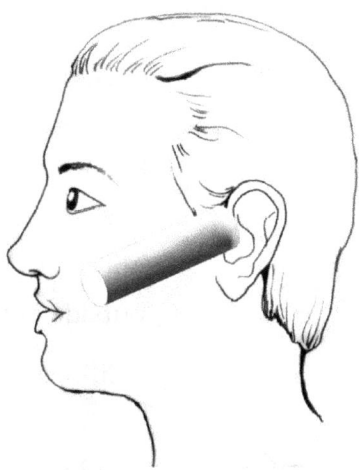

The highlight and shadow pattern in the cheek-bone area is similar to the cylinder. The illusion of a more defined cheek-bone can be created with the proper placement of the shadow and highlights.

MAKE UP

Application:

You want to first locate the lower area of the cheek-bone, which can be easily done using a finger. Beginning in the middle of the general area, and pressing gently, gradually moving along the cheek-bone. Notice that (arrow A) shows that there has been more of a depression or change created along the bottom line of the cheek-bone. This is the location where you will want to begin applying the shadow.

The area you will be working on is the cheek-bone, where it extends from the ear area to the corner of the eye. As in (arrow B) using your finger, move along the cheek-bone, until you have located the upper edge of it (arrow B), and begin applying the highlight in this area, following the edge of the hair to just the outside of the corner of the eye.

You may have some difficulties in locating the cheek-bone when working with a full shape face. In this case begin with the front of the cheek-bone, starting at the curve, following it backwards. You are going to find that the position of the cheek-bone, as well as the length, and width may vary in each individual.

MAKE UP

Camouflage, Concealers, Color Theory, and Counter Balance:

You will find that often there will be many different names referring to the same things. And you will come across a lot of them when dealing with corrective make-up. Eventually, you are going to encounter all of the different terms used regarding corrective make-up. When you have an area that isn't wanted, you are going to be using a camouflage made-up of concealers. The make-up artist will do this by creating an effect to counter balance the color that has already been used in the specific area.

Now, keeping that in mind we are going to refer to the product you will be using for this as a concealer for the rest of this section. In order to be successful at concealing areas that are a problem one needs a good understanding of the color theory, at least the basics of it. So for this area we are going to refer to the color wheel.

Remember, for the wheel of color for make-up there is going to be only three primary colors, and they are: Blue, Yellow, and Red. These three primary colors can stand on their own, and are used in the making all the other colors you will be using. Next, you are going to see that there are also three secondary colors: Orange, Violet, and Green. These are colors you get by combining two of the primary colors together.

MAKE UP

When you mix the primary colors of Red & Yellow you will get a secondary color of = orange.

When mixing primary colors of Red & Blue you will get a secondary color of = Violet.

When mixing primary colors of Yellow & Blue you will get a secondary color of = Green.

We will now continue with the intermediate colors, which are: Red-orange, Yellow-Orange, Yellow-Green, Blue-Green, Blue-Violet, and Red-Violet. You get these colors by combining a primary color with an already made secondary color.

About right now you are asking, how does this have anything to do with make-up? Well, that is because there are some colors that can be used to cancel out or rather, neutralize some of the other colors.

Examples of this would be:

If you needed to conceal the color blue, you would use orange.

To conceal red, you would use green.

And to conceal violet, you would use yellow.

The main purpose of using concealers is so that you can take a negative color issue and correct it. You will find these are areas that a make-up artist may encounter.

MAKE UP

Some of these negative problems while working on a face are:

Negative issues with blemishes. With this issue you will usually deal with the problem having to do with the color red. Useing a concealer which has green in it will cancel out the red.

Circles under the eyes will have issues with blue or violet colors, or blue/violet. Using a concealer that has orange in it will cancel out the blue, an a concealer that has yellow in it will cancel out violet.

Also, if you use a combination of orange and yellow you can cancel out a blue/violet color issue.

At times when you need to use concealers, you need to take into consideration the color of the skin. You will need to match the concealer as close to the skin color as possible, do not match the concealer to the shade of the discoloration.

When working with the eyes, and you are correcting violet or a dark blue color, remember to match the skins surrounding area, and not the area of the discoloration, rather, not the darkness within the discoloration. Otherwise, you will end up with dark circles that has been built up from the concealer. You want it to end up with violet and dark blue instead.

You will run into the same issues anytime you are

correcting acne or blemish discolorations. Sometimes a concealer can also be used as a shadow or highlighter, it depends on the shade and color. There is usually wax, or pigment that has a higher level of concentration, which can increase its coverage.

Depending on the amount and extent of and area to be corrected, you can apply the concealer before & after. Usually, one will apply the base first, then apply the concealer as needed, putting the concealer directly over the base. If you find some discoloration, or unevenness in the skin tone it can usually be dealt with in this matter.

Concealer should only be used if truly necessary, and then use a dab at a time, building up only as needed.

Application:

Once you have the base application, you will analyze the entire face. You do this in order to detect any negative problems with the colors. Looking carefully inside the corners of the eye, and under the eyes, now examine the face and neck for any blemishes that may be present. Now, using the color theory section of this lesson, decide which concealer matches the skin color, and will also counter balance the problem you are having with the color in general. Now choose either a small concealer brush, a sponge, or a small eye shadow brush to use for the

MAKE UP

application (noting that a brush is the most accurate).

In order not to remove any base that has been previously applied just use a tapping motion. Keep in mind, it is always best to use a small amount at a time, and add more when you need to. Now, take the sponge that you used to apply the base and gently roll it over the concealer area, blending the concealer into the base, be gentle, you do not want any of the product to stick to the sponge.

If you have a correction to do, and it is only a minor one, put some concealer onto a brush, and paint it gently over the area to be corrected. However, should it be a bigger problem, or if it is going to need a heavier application of concealer, use the flat side of the brush and gently pat the concealer onto the area that needs the correction. The patting motion is going to help in building up more of the product. Remember to only use what's necessary, especially in the area of the eyes, for too much will only create a messy look. Should there be a need for a heavier application keep tabs on it, because it could end up with creasing. Should too much creasing occur, continue to pat off the excess gently with the brush until the creases are eliminated, once they have been eliminated, powder the area.

MAKE UP

Chapter Study Questions

1. The study of Chiaroscuro is the study of what?

2. Is it possible for a make-up artist to correct all areas that have a problem?

3. Use orange to conceal what color?

4. What color is a blemish?

5. What are the factors to be used when choosing a concealer color?

6. Are shadows and highlights required for all nose corrections?

7. Is there a hard edge and a soft edge where you find wrinkles?

8. Is it best to use a lot of concealer when you are using it?

9. Does a shadow pattern that is soft edge to soft edge have any hard edges?

10. Is concealer required for all make-up jobs?

CHAPTER 3: Eyebrows

The make-up artist needs to be able to recognize the different styles of eyebrows. The make-up artist needs to be able to determine which of the brow shapes is best for each individual. The make-up artist should be able to balance out the eyebrows, giving the face a natural look, that's also flattering.

The make-up artist will be able to observe how changing the shape of the eyebrows is effecting the overall expression of the face. Does it make the eyes look more open? Or, more closed? Is it lifting up the facial features? Or, is it bringing them down? The make-up artist will be able to shape the eyebrows, making them appear natural.

Physical Features Of The Eyebrows

There is a saying that goes like this "The eyes are the window into the soul". This saying couldn't be closer to the truth than the truth itself.

MAKE UP

Arch Peak

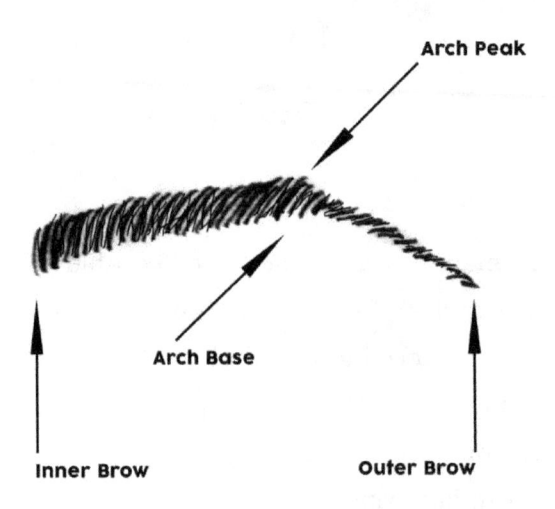

Arch Base

Inner Brow **Outer Brow**

There is a lot of work that goes into making-up a face, and the make-up artist will put forth much effort and time in doing their job. They have to spend time choosing what colors are needed, where to place the shadow, the position of the liner, which mascara to use, which brushes are best, they labor over their work just the way an artist of paintings do.

The artist of paintings would take time to choose the right frame to give his work enhancement, bringing out the best in the painting. A bad frame would take from its beauty, and with no frame it would leave the painting without any means of importance it seems.

We can say the same for the eyes. Without eyebrows, there is no life to the eyes. If the brows are badly shaped, or placed, it will take away from the eye appeal, as well as from the facial features them self.

Providing a frame for the upper eye, and consisting of a group of hairs, that grow just above the eyes, along the frontal-bone, is the eyebrows. Then there is the Zygomatic Arch (the upper cheek-bone),which provides the frame for the lower part of the face. When all this is put together, it lets the eye be the center point on the face.

When you take a good look at the face you will see that humans are not made to be symmetrical. You will hardly ever find two individuals with the same exact type of brows, each person's eyebrows will be different, it can range from a little bit different, to a lot different. A make-up artist can make one persons eyebrows look a lot like another, but unless they are identical twins, exact is not going to happen.

There are three parts to the eyebrow, they are: The outer brow, the inner brow, and the arch, which is the base and peak of the brow.

Placement Of The Classic Eyebrow

The shape of eyebrows in the 1900's and the difference in their shape today is astonishing. The brows had a sharper edge to them back then, however, they were considered to be classic, then and now.

MAKE UP

It is the job of the make-up artist to have the knowledge and be prepared to search for the most flattering brow shape for each individual they tend to. Both men and women need their brows groomed now and then, it helps to keep them well balanced.

Taking care of the brows, and giving them a shape, is a simple matter of adding too, or taking away from them. This is where (tweezing) comes into the picture. It's a simple matter of removing unwanted hair growth, and/or adding needed hair growth when necessary.

By shaping the brows you can give the face a totally different appearance. You can make the face appear to be sad, angry, or surprised, and so much more. Make the eyes closer together, or further apart.

It would seem that the options involved are infinite. It is up to the make-up artist to figure out which of the options should be used.

The benchmark position is one of standard measurement. And the classic eyebrow is called the touchstone. We will use this one in our lessons when talking about the placement of the eyebrows, and problems that can occur, as well as solutions to those problems.

All eyebrow shapes can be achieved from the basic position. This can be done by simply altering the brow. By altering, we are talking about changing the thickness or thinness of the brow. Changing the shape of the angle, and even giving the arch a little more roundness (changing the brow where it starts and ends).

The standard measurement of creating and positioning the eyebrow has seven basic steps. Use this as a guideline. Of course, this is in no way saying that everyone is going to have the same eyebrow shape. The shape of the eyebrows will vary, due to ones hair thickness or thinness, and there are some other things that will contribute to how ones shape turns out.

Some are going to be thin, while others will be more thicker. When determining which shape to use for a person you will start with the determining factors. The mystery of the eyebrow will be better understood once you understand these steps.

In determining the position of the eyebrow, you will go by several different parts of the eye itself. They are: The iris, the tear duct, the lower lid, the outside corner, and the upper lid.

Step 1

Inner Brow-Line

The inner brow-line is what determines where the

MAKE UP

eyebrow will begin (or the inside placement). This extends upward, beginning at the tear duct.

Step 2

Center-Line

The base and peak, or the arch and the center position will be determined by the use of the center-line, this extends upward, from the outside of the iris's edge.

Step 3

Outer Brow-Line

The inner brow-lines distance to the center-line is what determines the outer brow-line. This is approximately of equal distance to the outer brow-line from the base and peak (arch).

Step 4

Upper and Lower Lid-Lines

How wide the eye opens in-between the lower eye lid and the upper eye lid is what determines the horizontal positioning of the eyebrow itself.

MAKE UP

Step 5

Brow-Line

The brow-line is considered to begin one full "open eye" starting above the upper lash of that eye. This is where the brow-line should be.

Step 6

Arch Peak

The peak of the arch will be a full "open eye" starting at the base of the brow.

Step 7

The Arch's Base-Line

The base of the arch is about half the distance of the "open eye" going horizontally. And the height of the eyebrow is determined by the distance from the inner brow-line to the center.

Completed Classic Eyebrow

You have just went through the seven steps to the classic position of the eyebrow. Take note on the direction of hair growths in each of the sections of the graph.

MAKE UP

Growth Pattern Of The Classic Eyebrow

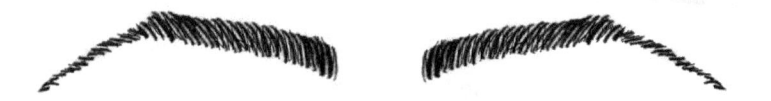

There is a growth pattern for eyebrows, they start at the inner eye-brow. The hairs in the eyebrows grow at the bottom of the brow first and grow upwards. The growth of the hair at the inner brow is angled slightly, and becomes even more angled as it gets closer to the arch. If you take notice, you will see that as you move along the brow each hair is slightly more angled then the preceding one.

When the hairs reach the arch the hairs become even more angled, and gradually start to get flat towards the outer brow.

Notice that the part of the brow that is the thickest is at the inner brow. Then the hairs begin to narrow as they start getting closer to the arch, and then taper off.

Usually, you'll find an equal distance between the hairs in the eyebrow. When you draw the eyebrow you should follow the growth pattern of the eyebrow itself. Begin with the inner-brow, continue up all the way to the arch, and end up at the outer-brow. This lets the make-up artist have a consistent pattern to go by. This can be used on anyone's eyebrow, it doesn't make any difference in the shape they desire.

Shaping the Eye-Brow

Since the face is not symmetrical both brows will rarely look identical. But, the idea of shaping them is not to make them look alike, but, as closely as they can be to looking alike. Giving them the appearance that they are equal in weight is why most people have them shaped. Others of course have them shaped for different reasons, the most popular reason would be for a more glamorous look.

MAKE UP

The space between the eyes should be the width of one eye. If the brows are too far apart the eyes appear to far apart, and if the brows are to close then it will give the appearance of the eyes being to close, giving the face an out of balanced look.

Sitting in as much natural light as possible face a mirror and take time to analyze the eyebrows. Examining both eyebrows for balance and positioning, and stay as objective as possible. Now, answer the questions that follow:

- Do the eyebrows appear over powering or heavy?
- Are the eyebrows too light and not hardly noticed?
- Are they flat, do the eyebrows have a good arch?
- Are the eyebrows without an arch, are they overly rounded?
- Does the space above the nose appear balanced, does the distance between the eye appear to far or to short?

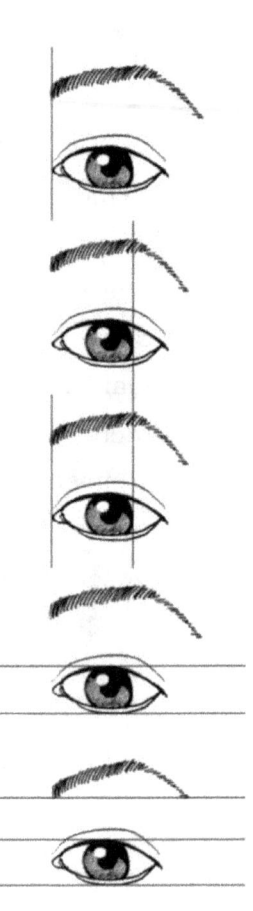

52

- Are the eyebrows full, or are there gaps or holes?
- Does the eyebrows have out of place hairs, any that stick up or out?
- Are both of the eyebrows at an equal height above the eyes?

All of these issues can be resolved by shaping the eyebrows.

Correcting Eyebrow Shapes

The shape of one's eyebrows can definitely make them give off a different expression, it can be either in a negative or a positive way.

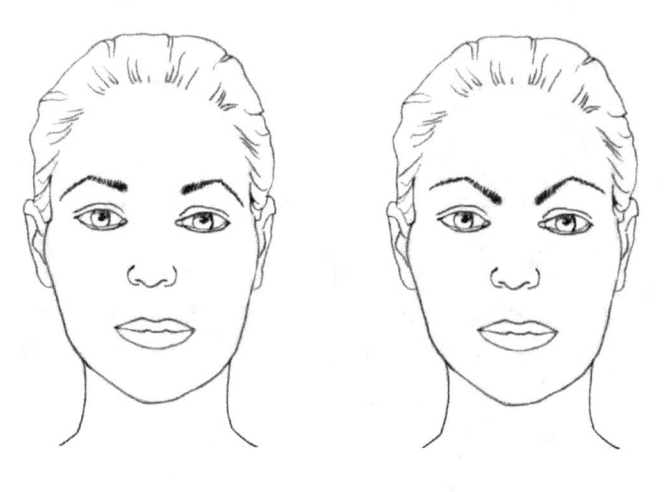

Illustration A   Illustration B

Notice in Illustration (A) the eyebrows are very thin and tend to make the eyes look un-framed. And in Illustration

MAKE UP

(B) the eyebrows are too heavy and tend to make the eyes and face appear weighed down.

Example:

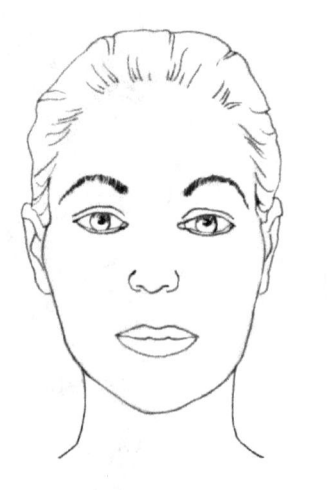

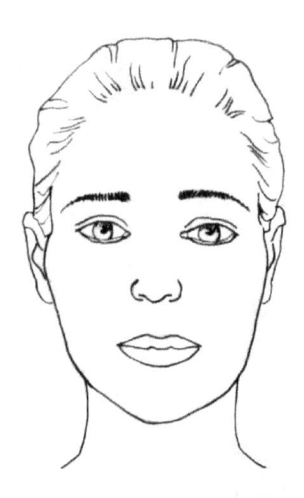

In (Illustration A) above the person's expression appears to be sad. It is because the eyebrows are slanting downward on the outer edge, giving the appearance of sadness.

Example:

In (Illustration B) above it gives the expression that they are angry. This is because the eyebrows are slanting downward on the inner edge.

MAKE UP

Illustration A   Illustration B

Example:

In (Illustration A) above the eyebrows have a very rounded appearance, so it gives the expression of being surprised.

Example:

In (Illustration B) above the person has an expression of being worried or perplexed. This is because the eyebrows have a flat appearance.

MAKE UP

CHAPTER 4:
Eye-Shadow

Applied properly, eye shadow will enhance one's eye's, and give them an outgoing perspective on things. Because it makes them feel more positive about themselves. The make-up artist is going to learn the benefits you can get from shadows and highlights when applying them as make-up on the eyes, and what the difference is in the two when you are using the shadow and highlights application.

It is the make-up artists job to be able to apply eye shadow on a face that is going to draw attention (in a good way). The make-up artist will be able to notice when there is a problem, and be able to correct it. The make-up artist should be able to correct a variety of problematic areas that show up with the eyes. The make-up artist will learn how to properly position the eye shadow in ways to enhance the facial features. To apply eye shadow to make someone's face look as though it has had a lift, by lifting the eye. They will also be able to create someone's face to give them a more youthful appearance.

MAKE UP

Physical Features Of The Eye

The area just above the eye, above the eye lid, (or directly under the eyebrow), is the area that eye shadow is usually wore. The height, and width of this area will vary in different individuals. Sometimes however, if the dramatic look is wanted, then the eye shadow may also be placed in different areas located around the eye, such as under, or around the outside corner.

This particular area has been taken apart and put into sections, which are:

- The lower eye lid.
- The upper eye lid.
- The brow-bone.
- The fold.
- The tear duct.
- The outer corner.

MAKE UP

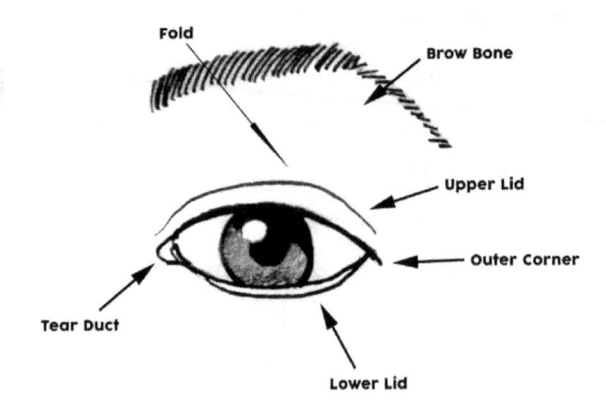

Eye diagram with labels: Fold, Brow Bone, Upper Lid, Outer Corner, Lower Lid, Tear Duct

The skin in this area will be loose in some individuals, while tight in other individuals. The more mature, or older person may have some uneven surfaces in their eye lids, eye lids such as this are commonly referred to as the eye lid with a creepy look about it. The younger people will have more youthful skin that appears to have a glow to them, and will be taut, and smooth.

Folds Of The Eye

Eyes are going to come in many different types, as well as shapes, having different types of folds in them. They can also be an oval shape, and sometimes you will find them rounded, and even in all of the various shapes they are going to come in, you are going to see many different types of folds in each of them. The area found under the brow to the top of the lid line, will be the part of the face that the make-up artist is going to focus on while applying eye-shadow.

The categories for the folds are as follows:

Slight fold

Flat fold

Heavy fold

Recessed eye

Asian heavy fold

Asian slight fold

Keep in mind that a fold can consist of a combination of any in the above list, or it can be only one. The make-up artist can create an illusion by using the correct positioning of the eyes shadow. Any of the folds or shapes can be altered with the eye shadow, and by using the shadow to pull down or lift up on the fold or shape, an illusion can be created, giving the appearance of a look that isn't actually there.

For instance, by diminishing the folds weight, you can create the illusion that the heavy fold is merely a light fold, and this is going to make the eyes appear as though they have been lifted up a lot more. Also the eyes will appear to be opened more. Naturally, this is going to give the entire face the appearance of having a face lift. If it is an older individual, it will also give the face a more youthful appearance.

The illustrations of the folds being referred to in this chapter can be found throughout this section. The illustrations will consist of the general fold types. Although, there will be a few folds that are exact, and even some that are from a combination of folds. It doesn't matter because, when the make-up artist is applying eye shadow, the basic principles will still apply.

Eye Shadow Placement

In order for the make-up artist to bring balance to the eyes, and gradually to the entire face, the process of putting on eye shadow applications will be used. This is done once the base has been applied, and the eyebrows are complete. The make-up artist will determine where to place the products by allowing the eyes to be framed by the eyebrows.

The outcome of applying the product depends on how, and where the product is applied. This is of the utmost importance, because the technique used also depend on how and where the product is applied for the outcome effect.

MAKE UP

Skin Care

A good application of eye shadow will be determined by the shape the skin is in. The skin's condition is an important factor to a good application. The area just above the eye should be cleaned good, and also moisturized properly before attempting to put on an application of eye shadow. An individual should keep their facial skin cleansed and moisturized on a daily basis. If this area is left unattended, the skin not only becomes rough and dried out, but can also have acne and blemishes appear.

If the make-up artist tries to apply eye shadow onto skin that hasn't been taken care of properly the application can turn out to be uneven, making it nearly impossible to get the colors blended together correctly, and the effect it should have may be spoiled.

Blending

Blending the eye shadows is something that needs to be done with great care. The blending of eye shadows is an art, and the make-up artist will need to take precautions in order to have a flawless edging, yet still have the smooth equality. The transition of colors will have to be kept flowing smoothly into one another when going from one color to a different color in a way that there is no big detection in the change.

MAKE UP

The difference in an average application, and a great application, is going to be noticeable by the brush that you use. It is important that you use a different brush for each of the colors you use. Should you get the brushes mixed up, even though there may not be any noticeable colors showing. It is possible that there could be just a tiny amount in the brush somewhere. And that tiny amount can make a big difference in the effect of the coloring. Among one of the worst things that could happen would be for the coloring to come out with a muddy looking effect.

So, keeping that in mind, along with blending cautiously, you now have the keys to a beautiful eye-shadow application.

Shadow and Highlight

The make-up artist must have an understanding about the things eye shadow can do for a person's eyes before attempting to apply. Shadow and highlights are the two most important key elements in the application of eye shadow.

The difference in the color when it comes to the shadows and the highlights is in the shading. Take the shading in shadows for instance, the shading in shadows will be darker in color, whereas the shading in highlights is going to be a bit lighter in color. The shadow and the

MAKE UP

highlights will each serve a different purpose during the make-up application.

When looking for a color that works good with all different colors of eyes, and will also match well for skin tones, most of them anyway. Just keep in mind that neutral colors can work with all eye colors, and make note that when using neutral colors , make-up with the natural look works best. These would include taupe, and brown (warm ones such as light brown). And the highlight that works best on any eye color would be the soft yellow, or a cream that is of a very light color.

If you want to draw attention to a certain area, you can do so by using a highlight in order to make that area appear to be enhanced or stand out. Shadows will make an area appear to be pushed backwards, creating more depth. When used in combination, eyes that appear unbalanced can be balanced out using this technique. Much like the outer fold and the tired eye.

Where you place the shadows and highlights will depend on the particular fold of the eye area because each of the folds has their own special requirements. The reason for us to apply the highlight first is so that we will have a template to go by when applying the shadow. That is because when applying the highlight it leaves an area behind (which we will call a template), and this is a big help in guiding us when we apply the shadow.

MAKE UP

Although each fold has its individual requirements, we can also use the common elements which most folds will apply too. Never put the eye-shadow on past the outside corner and lift up on the lid at all times when applying the shadow. The reason for this is due to the effect it will have on the eye, which would be weighting it down and give the appearance of drooping.

It is important for the make-up artist to remember and always take time to blend the edges well, if it doesn't get blended good it can leave it looking harsh and sloppy. So always blend them well, giving the appearance of having a soft edge.

In general, the eye-shadow will not be put on any lower than the tear duct (on the inside edge). This will also leave an after effect that makes the eye appear to be drooping. Except when the make-up artist is working with Asian eyes, due to the shape of Asian eyes it may be beneficial to apply just a little past the tear duct.

Notice how the following examples give eye-shadow positioning, with placement for correcting. For instance; the Asian Slight Fold has three different choices of use, and the Asian Heavy Fold has the ability to take elements from the three Asian Slight Folds choices and adapt them for its needs.

Whichever way the make-up artist goes about it, each

is going to have their unique ending effect. It is of great importance and most beneficial for the make-up artist to remember "Shadows Push" and "Highlights Pull."

Use the following examples that show the placement of eye-shadow when corrections apply:

The Flat Eye

The shape of this eye is a little bit concaved. It is referred to as flat due to the fact that it has no noticeable imperfections. The perfect shaped eye gives the make-up artist plenty of ground to explore and experiment with different extraordinary eye-shadow treatments.

The Slight Fold (Above)

When working with the slight fold the make-up artist will only need to do minor corrections to make the eyes look more glamorous, and appear more open. Should there be a need to put a little more dimension towards the shadow it will be necessary to put a little highlighter on the upper eye lid, and also the brow-bone.

Recessed Eye

Having almost no fold at all is referred to as the recessed eye. It will be necessary to pin point the area on the bone just below the brow, finding the area that protrudes away from the eye the most. This is where the shadow will be placed. Whether or not there is

going to be any highlighter under the brow will depend on how much space is available for it.

Heavy Fold

When working with an eye that has a heavy fold, look for the area on the lid where the skin is hanging at its heaviest point. Now, by applying the highlighter and shadow in this area it is going to create a younger appearance, and give the illusion it has been lifted.

Asian Slight-Fold (1)

The shape of this eye is much less pronounced than other eyes. In general, this eye is shaped like an Asian eye (known as the Imposed Caucasian), whereas it usually isn't very pronounce. Take notice where the fold is hanging over the lid (by the degrees). Giving an appearance to the eye lid that it is flat. By using some shadow and highlights on the eye lid it can give it more dimension, and give it the illusion of appearing more rounded, and it will appear to be more open.

MAKE UP

Asian Slight-Fold (2)

The dimension can be crafted to be just a little bit different than the other one, giving the appearance that the eye is open somewhat more than in the previous illustration. This is a good position to use for this shape, and also this type of fold.

Asian Slight-Fold (3)

The make-up artist can give this shape a little dimension with a vertical angle by placing shadows and highlights on the outer area and the inner area of the lid.

Asian Heavy-Fold

Having a flat appearance like the Asian Slight-Fold, and the heaviness of the fold hiding the lid itself. Most of the time in cases such as this, the eye lashes are going downward.

The make-up artist can change the heavy fold area giving it more balance, which is going to make it appear to be more rounded.

Take Note:

The three Asian positions in the above illustrations will

MAKE UP

all work with the Asian Heavy-Fold.

Remember:

The illustrations of positions above are based on the types in general of the different folds that the make-up artist may encounter. If you refer to the illustrations found in the "Basic Principles Of Highlights, Balance & Shadows" you'll see that it is also possible to have a combination of the folds.

Illustrations Of Shadow Placements

Below you will find some illustrations on placements for shadows to apply on the eye lids (opened and closed).

Take a good look at how the shadows are being blended in with the highlights. You will be able to see the difference between the hard and soft edges with these illustrations. This will be the shadows soft edge blending with the highlights soft edge. Remember in the beginning of our lessons, we learned that the shadow doesn't usually get placed on the eye lid any farther than its corner.

There is a noticeable difference between the folds with shadows and highlights and the folds without anything on them at all (illustrations above).

The make-up artist can make the appearance of the

MAKE UP

folds seems flawless when using the proper amount of product, along with good blending techniques. Mastering the application of applying beauty make-up is a necessity in blending shadows and highlights properly.

Illustrated Positions With "Asian Folds"

The Flat-Eye (1)   **Asian Slight-Fold**

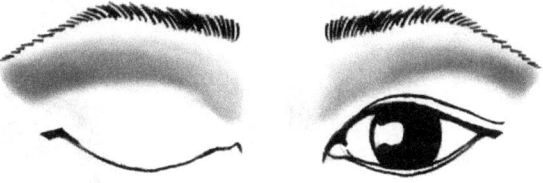

The Slight-Fold (2)   **Asian Slight-Fold**

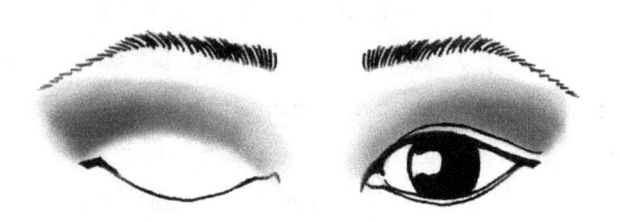

The Recessed-Eye-Fold (3)   **Asian Slight-Fold**

MAKE UP

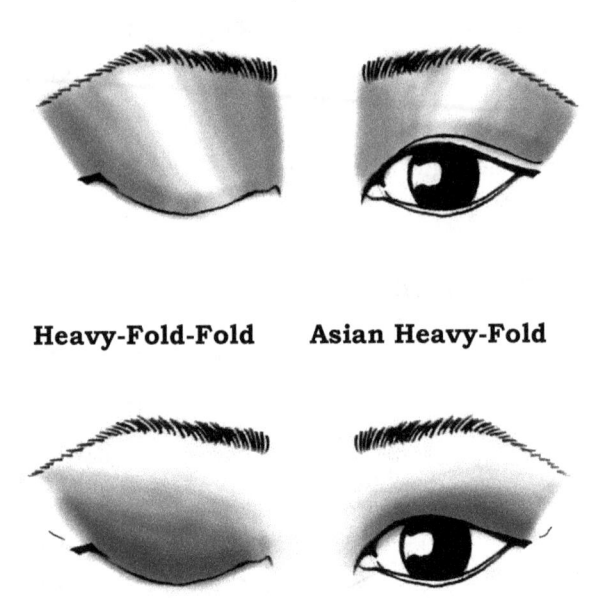

Heavy-Fold-Fold   Asian Heavy-Fold

Remembering that not every eye will be symmetrical. However, the same person is capable of having more than one fold , and they may even have a combination/variation of one or more of the folds here in the example illustrations. Now it is time for an assessment of the eyes.

You will need to pick out which brush that you are going to use for highlighting (one of your little eye-brush ones will work just fine). You are now ready to start building your product using little dabs at a time, building by increments, which is what works best. This way it lets

MAKE UP

the make-up artist keep control of the situation, and it also will help the make-up artist ensure that it stays in balance, and even during the application.

Letting the product build up by increments will benefit you, as it will help keep the product from layering in a bulky matter, or dripping all over the place. If you are working with dark colors building up a bulky mess will not be a good thing, and unprofessional. Not to mention if it should drip all over the mess you'll have.

Another reason to do it by increments would be to avoid getting it on the model's face and have to remove all the previous work, and start it completely over. It would consist of removing all excess product, and other stuff such as foundation. Next, you would start over by re-applying the base, then the shadows and highlights, and after all that you have re-apply the foundation, and of course the eye-shadow.

Load The Brush

When you go to load your brush you want to let the product slowly build up on the brush. To do this simply tap the brush lightly, as you are dipping it in the eye-shadow. The product can be distributed more evenly if the brush is loaded on both sides.

Always start out the application using a little of the

product at a time, re-loading the brush when necessary in order to build it up onto the eye in small increments. If the make-up artist uses techniques like this it gives them the choice of how much to use, how to go about loading, and how much to build it up.

The make-up artist should go by what they have learned in these lessons, practicing until they have mastered all of the different situations encountered. Thereby, preventing re-moving, and re-starting the application process over and over.

Where To Place The Highlights

Begin the application process by placing the highlight over the brow-bone area just below the eye-brow. Give the brush a few soft and light strokes (you can also use the tapping motion if you prefer) and place the highlight.

You will be working from the inside out, upward towards the arch, and ending at the outer corner of the brows edge. Do not lift the brush while in the process of your blending application, instead swipe the brush from one side of the eye-lid to the other, in a back and forth motion.

The make-up artist will ask the model to close their eyes while applying the application, continue with the process moving from the inside corner near the tear duct and going across the eye-lids middle, all the way to the other side. Finishing on the outer side, in the corner.

Being careful not to go past the outside edge of the eyes corner, leaving an after effect that makes the eye appear to be dropping. You will be putting the highlight on all the way to where the fold meets with the upper lid. Next, it's time to begin the application process with the eye-shadow!

Where To Place The Shadow

For this part of the application you need an eye-shadow brush of medium size. Having the model face downward, and lightly stroke (or use a tapping motion again, if you like) and place the eye-shadow into the fold area. Now and then you will ask the model to look straight ahead in order to examine your placement. The part of the fold that is the heaviest is where you will be placing the shadow.

The shadow is used in this area to push the folds back, these folds are a distraction and give unwanted effects such as a drooping appearance. Blending edges from shadow to highlights working with the fold. This technique is combining the soft edge to the soft edge.

If the make-up artist decides to use the drop shadow to enhance the models lashes it is done by creating an illusion that they are so long that they cast their own shadow. This is at times used in order to balance a upper eye issue having an effect of being too heavy.

To do a drop shadow the make-up artist will place a drop of shadow on the lower eye-lid (under the lower lashes). It is best to ask the model to look upward while doing this application.

For the eyes drop shadow, the wedge shaped angle brush should be used, but a small eye shadow brush will do the trick. Now you will make gentle strokes going across the lower lid, continue blending in as you go. The blending should take place all the way across the lid, with the model still looking straight ahead.

Keep an eye in a mirror, and always check work before moving on. Then adjust whenever it is necessary.

Glamour And Fashion

Variety can be added by using the available techniques that is going to allow for elaboration, letting you create with neutral tones, giving a dramatic appearance to the make-up and eye treatment.

A well blended application is of utmost importance, of course, the shades of the shadows used are equally important to get a well blended application. Neutral shades if applied correctly can be used to enhance, and even

MAKE UP

change the appearance of the eyes.

The effect depends on the shades that are used, and how well they get blended. The make-up artist can even choose to use shadows that involve numerous shades. Should this be the case, the application will begin using the lightest to the darkest shades of shadow.

This is another one of those procedures that lets you build up by increments, with the make-up artist having control of the dimensions and final effect.

The following examples will show the different appearances that can be created when adding shadows in layers. Usually, this will start with the lightest shade, and end with the darker shade.

With each new layer it will progress dramatically. You can go with any of the following looks, whatever you decide you want from the ending effect.

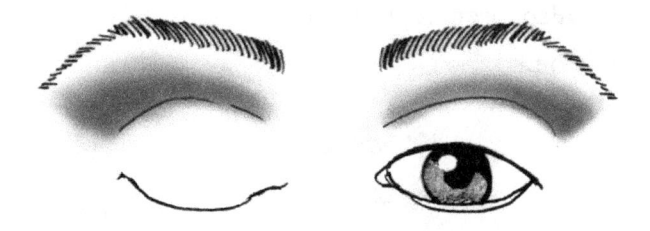

Example One

The positioning for an eye that is flat, is the standard

MAKE UP

shadow positioning. Strangely enough, it just happens to be the base that treatments of other shadows begin from. A highlight is placed on the eye-lid, under the eye-brow, and a taupe shade of shadowing is positioned.

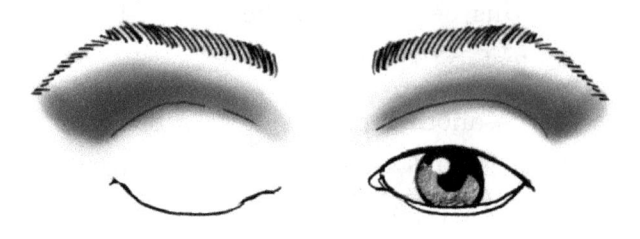

Example Two

In this treatment with the eye shadow the lid space have been narrowed by bringing the shadow slightly down onto the lid. It begins with a shade of taupe, and each color thereafter is just slightly darker in color. This helps in giving more depth in the appearance of the eye. There has also been a little highlight placed on the brow-bone and the lid.

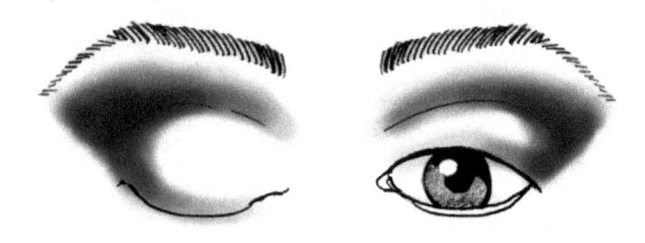

MAKE UP

Example Three

For this treatment you apply the shadow around the eye and then apply the highlights in layers. The color of the shades will be best in appearance if they are blended in to the shadows starting with the lightest shade and ending with the darkest shade (the darker shades works best when blended into the fold).

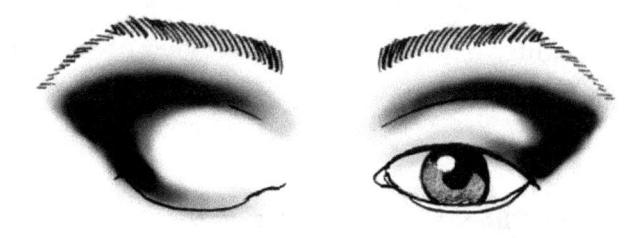

Example Four

Similar to the treatment above, but there has been a shadow of black added over the dark brown, and then well blended. Careful not to let the brush get excess dark colors in it.

MAKE UP

CHAPTER 5:
Cheeks

It is important to use the proper technique for the application process of applying the cheek color. You want this to appear natural. If properly done it will enhance the finished make-ups appearance, and add life to it as well.

The make-up artist will be able to choose the proper colors for the cheeks, this includes the base, shadows, highlights, and foundation, and let's not forget about the rouge for the cheek-bones.

The Cheeks Physical Features

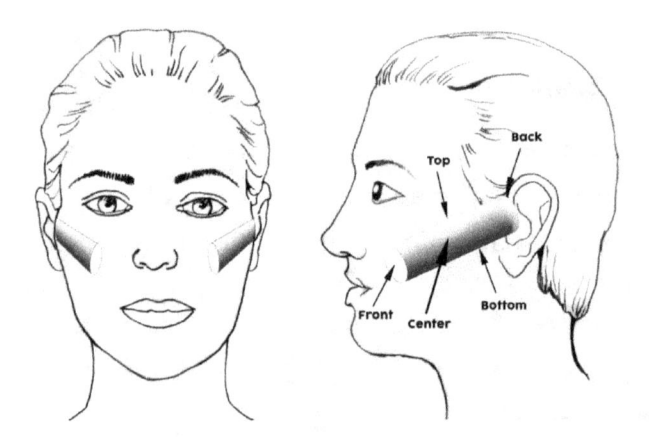

The cheek-bone is the frame for the eyes as well as the entire face. Referencing back to the chapter on eyebrows,

MAKE UP

you'll notice that the eye is using the eyebrows as its upper frame. Attention will be drawn to the facial features once dimension is added by applying color to the cheek bones, ultimately providing a lift to the face.

The cheekbone is located on the side of the face between the corner of the eye and the earlobe. The technical term for cheekbone id Zygomatic Arch. Notice how there is a depression under the cheekbone, this is where the cheekbone starts to naturally curve inward.

The areas of the cheekbones will be referred to in this chapter as follows:

The area where the cheekbone begins is in front of the cylinder.

The area where the cylinder ends is in the back, at the center of the ear.

The highlight is placed where the light hits the highest part on the cheekbone, which is on top of the cylinder.

The shadow is placed where the cheek begins to curve inward, this is located at the bottom of the cheekbone.

Cheek color is placed in the center of the cheekbone. This is the area between the base of the cylinder and the top of it.

MAKE UP

Where To Position The Cheek Color

Once the eye treatments are complete the make-up artist will then continue with the cheek area. The use of a cheek color brush is used in applying Blush or cheek color to the cheeks. The cheek color brush is specially made, and will assist in creating a natural enhancing effect.

Apply the cheek color to the cheek-bone moving along the length of the cheek, and centered. This is the cylinders mid tone area, beginning at the hair follicle and ending at the corner of the eye, the area where the curve of the cheek-bone curves upward.

Referring to the shadows and highlights section regarding the cheek-bone of the corrective makeup chapter, it is possible for the make-up artist to apply the shadows and highlights during the base application.

Color Products For The Cheeks

There are several product types available for cheek colors, with cream and powder products being on the top of the list. Cheek color gels are becoming more popular, which tend to be more translucent than cream or powder products that only produce a simple hint of color.

When you are using a powder cheek color, it is important that your model is powdered adequately.

MAKE UP

Powdering is the last step of applying foundation. If it is needed, additional powder may be lightly applied before you apply cheek color.

Powder will simply slide over powder, which ensures a well blended and smooth application. If the model isn't powdered correctly, the cheek color could adhere to the skin and leave blotches of color on the cheeks.

When it comes to using cream cheek color, the make-up artist will powder after the cheek color is applied. This will become part of the process of building the foundation.

Cheek color gel is normally used when powdering isn't needed, keeping the application translucent.

Powder Cheek Color

In order to load your brush, gently swipe a blush brush back and forth across the powder blush. Tap into a clean tissue in order to remove any excess powder from the brush.

Application

Begin at the back of your cheekbone towards the hairline. Gently place the brush upon the skin.

MAKE UP

Using small circular motions, even moving your brush from the back of the cheekbone towards the front. If you are wanting more color, just re-apply. It is easier to build color from light to more intense, than to lighten a intense color after too much product has been applied to skin.

Don't bring the powder color too far to the front of the cheekbone. Simply, stop at the corner of the eye. Cheek color should not drop below the nostrils.

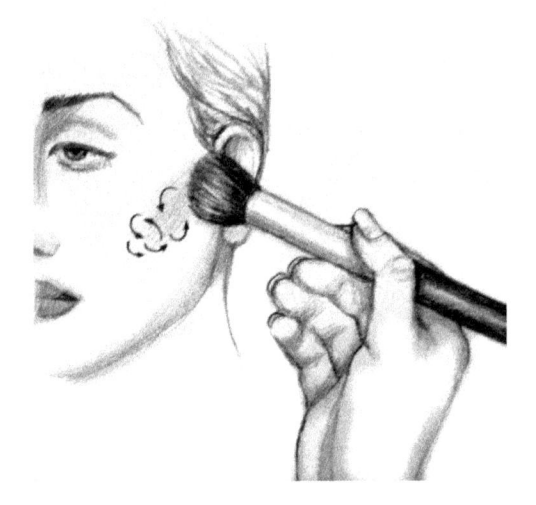

Cream Cheek Color

Most of the same principles of applying powder cheek color will apply to cream cheek color. There are a few important differences that an artist should take note of.

Cream cheek color is great for those who have dry skin or when a sheet of color is wanted.

MAKE UP

Due to the amount of slip, those who have oily skin should not use cream cheek colors. The same goes for the placement of cream cheek color. The difference is the application or sequence and the tools that are used to apply it with.

Cream cheek color should be applied before you powder. There is a simple reason for this, think about cream to cream type of products. If you are wanting a well blended, smooth application, the cream cheek color will need to go on an non-powdered foundation application. Cream will adhere to another cream product. If you have already powdered a model's face, cream cheek color will adhere and then streak along the cheekbone. This type of combination will not give you smooth blending.

Application

The placement area for the cream cheek color will be the same as using a powder cheek color. Begin from the back of the cheekbone and work your way forward or begin on the center of the cheekbone.

Cream cheek application may be done with your fingers, brush, or sponge.

After you have selected the correct cheek color for your model, remove a small amount of the product with a palette knife. Place your product onto your make-up

MAKE UP

palette, and use a sponge/brush. Smooth any lumps that may be in the make-up by tapping the brush/sponge back and forth on a clean area of you make-up palette. Begin with the placement of the cheek color near the model's hairline and smooth it forward going towards the nose. Remember it is easy to build intensity than it is to having too much product and having to completely remove it because it is too much. Be sure that the edges of the cheek color are smooth and well blended and that there are no streaks. When you use your fingers to apply, start with tapping the product on the center of your cheekbone and gently blend with a light stroking type motion.

Gel Cheek Color

Gel cheek colors are mostly transparent and will create a wash color. This is nice when the make-up has a real make-up feel and only needs a hint of color.

When you are using gel as a cheek color, it is always best to not have any powder on the make-up application. The powder will certainly clump when it is mixed with a gel. Cheek gels that are water-based will dry quickly and are not recommended for models who have dry skin. Other cheek gels that are not water-based, but will work great on a dry skin.

In order to apply, please refer to the application section

of cream cheek color.

Selecting Color and The Natural Look

In order to select a cheek color that looks natural on a model's skin, simply follow the guidelines below:

The lighter the skin, the lighter the shades should be.

Use colors like apricot, soft pink, rose, and light peach on fair skin tones.

Medium skin tones can wear warm rose, coral, plum and soft beige.

Dark skin will need a deeper and intense color in order to be seen on the skin. Use a rust, dark plum, deep brick, berry, and orange colors on dark skin.

Highlight Colors

When you are selecting the highlight color, be sure that it is in the same color family as the cheek color. Although, the highlight color will need to be at least 2 or 3 shades lighter. Eye shadow as well as a cheek color may be used for this process. Extremely light skin can be highlighted using pale shades of eye shadow as long as they are within the same colors of the cheek color. For example, when you use soft apricot as the cheek color and then your highlight color should be a pale yellow or peach that is used along

MAKE UP

the top of the cheekbone in order to highlight it.

Shadow Colors

In order to accent the base of your cheekbone, the shadow color should be at least 2 or 3 shades deeper than the color that has been chosen for the center of the cheek bone. Powder eye shadow can be used in order to accent the base of your cheekbone, if the cheek color doesn't offer a variety of deep shades.

For those who have dark skin, powder eye shadows like deep, warm brown can be used to shade the cheekbone if a rust or brick cheek color has been used on the cheekbone.

Whatever color or product you have selected, it will remain necessary to blend all areas of the application.

Common Cheek Color Mistakes

Application Mistake:

The color placed on the cheek has made it appear too far out.

MAKE UP

Effect:

If you bring the cheek color too far forward on the face, it will give an effective of having the face pulled down.

On a natural thin face, there may be very defined cheekbones and it will need to be shaded. Bringing the cheek color too far forward can cause the cheekbones to look more hollow, which will cause the face to look more gaunt.

A very full face that doesn't have well defined cheekbones, if the cheek color goes too far forward it will cause the focus of the face downward. This causes the face to have an illusion of jowls and that isn't flattering and not the purpose of using cheek color.

Application Mistake:

The placement of the blush is too high.

Effect:

If the cheek color is too high and is placed on the top of the cheekbone where the highlight should be, it will have a flattening effect on the face. Instead of the cheek color being in the center of the cheekbone to give it dimension, the color will diminish the balance that is trying to be created.

MAKE UP

Application Mistake:

The placement of Blush is too low.

Effect:

If the color is placed too low, by placing the color on the bottom of the cheekbone, it will have an effect of lowering the natural cheekbone. This will distort the perception of the placement of the cheekbone and will cause the look to be unbalanced.

Application Mistake:

More than enough blush has been applied.

Effect:

If there is too much cheek color on the cheekbone, it will overwhelm the face. The true goal of applying natural cheek color is to bring a natural warmth and glow to the skin. Too much color can cause the skin to look garish

Application Mistake:

Not enough color has been applied to the cheek area.

MAKE UP

Effect:

If there isn't enough cheek color on the cheekbone will defeat the purpose of ever applying the cheek color.

Application:

The cheek color has not been blended very well.

Effect:

If the edges of the cheek color are not blended correctly, it will have a striped result instead of a diffused, soft blend along the cheekbone. If you are wanting a smooth, natural and even looking application, remember to swirl the blush brush along the cheekbone in light, soft circles. This simple technique will help to ensure that there aren't any harsh edges in the cheek color application.

Chapter Study Questions

1. What are the terms used for cheek color?
2. The cheek-bone resembles what geometric shape the most?
3. What area of the cheek-bone would you apply cheek color?

MAKE UP

4. Does cheek color only come in powder form?

5. Are color gels more translucent or less translucent?

6. What is the name of the brush use to apply powder cheek color?

7. What type of motion is used to apply the powder cheek color?

8. What area do you place the highlighter when working with the cheek-bone?

9. What are of the cheek-bone do you place the shadow?

10. Which would you apply to the cheek-bone, a hard edge or a soft edges?

CHAPTER 6:
Lips

Using the appropriate application when applying lip color will help to maintain the balance, and proportions of the lips. The application of color to the lips is usually the final process in applying beautiful make-up. If it is done correctly, it will bring everything together and complete your make-up, and giving it a highlighted appearance. In this chapter, the make-up artist is going to learn the techniques of applying color to the lips, including how to outline the lips to make corrections to irregular shaped lips and add definition. Irregular lip shapes can include uneven, drooping, even thin or oversized lips.

PHYSICAL FEATURES OF THE LIPS

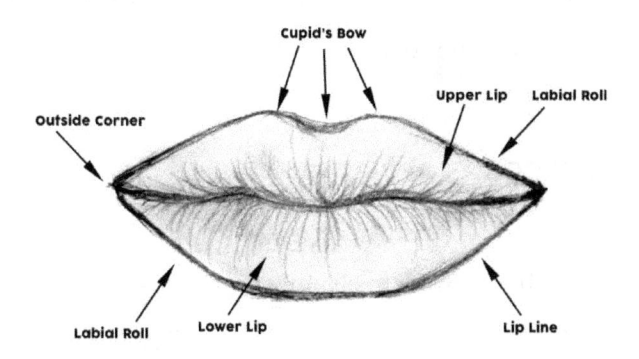

MAKE UP

Lips are made of tissues that are soft and pliable, generally with a defined edge know as the lip line which surrounds the both the upper and lower lip. The line of the lip helps determine the end of the lips.

Upper lips will generally have two high points and a valley called the Cupid's bow in the center, however it can be different from one person to the next. The cupid's bow may be higher, pointed, rounded, and some do not have a Cupid's bow.

The labial roll is a characteristic that circles the lips edge, and brings additional dimensions and definition to the lips. The labial roll can be extremely noticeable on some people, and hardly noticed on others. The width and color tone of the persons skin can have an impact on the appearance as well. Without the naturally occurring highlight, the lips will appear flat and have no dimension.

As you read this chapter, there will be references regarding the corners of the mouth where the upper, and lower lips come together.

LIP COLOR APPLICATION

Prior to applying color to the lips, the make-up artist should have knowledge and a good understanding about the various products used. There are many products the artist can choose from, such as cream or matte lip color, even tinted lip gloss. There are even various application methods available, from lipstick to pots like lip gloss.

The cream applications will usually have some type of moisture which helps keep the product moist. Benefits of this include easy application, and being better on the lips if they are dried, rough, or even chapped compared to other options.

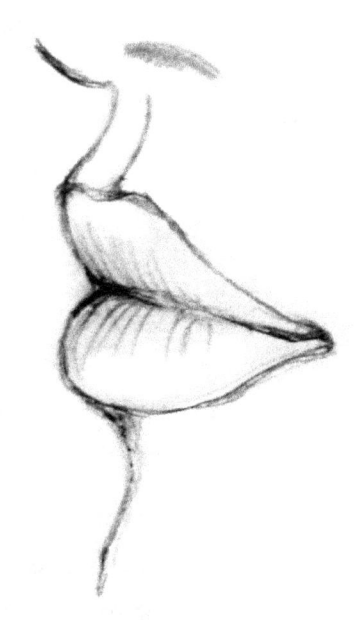

A matte lip color product is usually much dryer than the alternative cream products and have very little, if any shine to them. Because they are naturally a dryer product, this means it will often stay better and last longer.

With the application of adding lip color, it's just as it

sounds, applying color to the lips using the best product for the situation. Applying color to the lips helps the overall make-up process as it adds more features and draws attention to the mouth region. Because adding color to the lips is often the last step in the make-up process, it is what finishes off the look.

Prior to applying any lip color product, you should take notice to the condition of the lips. The health of lips is also important when choosing which product to apply. Aiming for a smooth and easy application process is the goal for defining the lip line edges. For a good application, the lips should be in good condition and smooth. Rough or chapped lips will result in the applied color also being rough and uneven. Because of this, the lips can be exfoliated and moisturized just like the skin to help keep them in healthy condition. This will help them from drying out, chapping and being rough.

Lips can be moisturized on a daily basis, and exfoliated when needed. Because the tissues of the lips are quite sensitive it's important not to over-exfoliate. You may find using a scrub created for exfoliating is helpful, and a moisturizing cream can help with the dryness.

Like coloring between the lines, adding color to the lips is done between the lip lines to create a natural looking and defined appearance. The following image provides an example of how lips appear once the lip color has been applied.

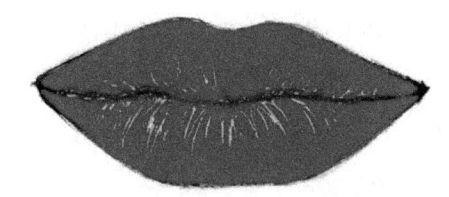

Loading a lipstick brush is one of the first, and essential application methods a make-up artist has to learn. There are various ways the artist can transfer color from the lipstick tube, to the brush.

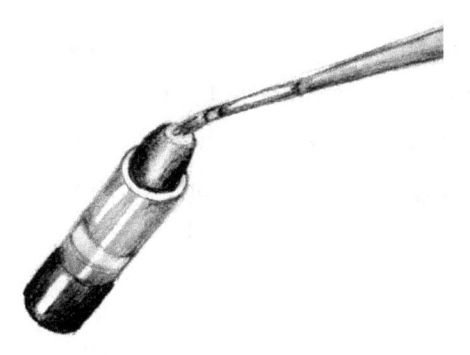

One of the methods includes transferring the color straight from the lipstick tube, to the brush. However, it's suggested to only use this method if the person owns the lipstick tube and not if it is shared with anyone else.

An alternative method includes using a palette knife.

MAKE UP

Simply use it to remove small portions of color from the tube, and transfer it to a palette or other surface. You may then transfer the color to a brush. The use of a brush will help provide definition and hard edges to the lip line.

You can load the lip brush by moving the brush through the color, similar to an artist getting paint on his brush using a back and forth motion. The brush should be nearly flat when moving across the color, this promotes an even coat on each side of the brush. Take caution that you are not causing the brush to rub, or mash into the color product because this will damage the brush's bristles and give you an uneven application.

Once you have got color on your brush using the best application you should have the model slightly open her mouth and give a smile. This causes the lips to tighten, making it easier to provide an cleaner, and sharper application.

MAKE UP

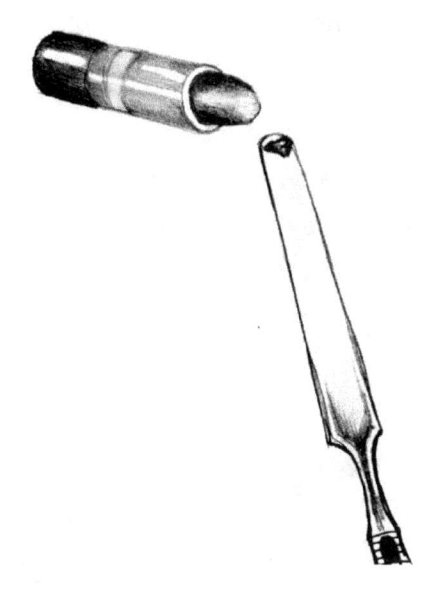

UPPER LIP

Start on the outside corner, position the brush flat on the lip so the brush edge is against the lips edge.

Move the brush in and upward motion, go in the direction of the Cupid's bow. Once you hit the peak, move the brush downwards and continue to follow the lips edge toward the center of the lip.

Turn brush over, this side should have color. Continue on opposite side of models mouth.

Reload your brush.

LOWER LIP

MAKE UP

Start with the flat part of the brush against the outer corner of lip, continue to follow lip edge. Drag brush to center and stop.

Repeat the same steps from other side of mouth, again stop when you reach the center.

Request model to close her mouth, fill any additional areas with color product.

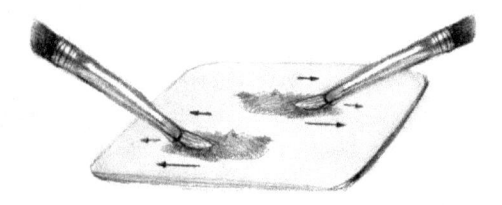

Note:

Keep the strokes of your brush continuous so they flow together. Once you begin, don't lose contact, it's important to keep consistent amounts of pressure on your brush to get an even application of color on the lips. You should attempt to cover each lip with no more than two strokes of the brush.

MAKE UP

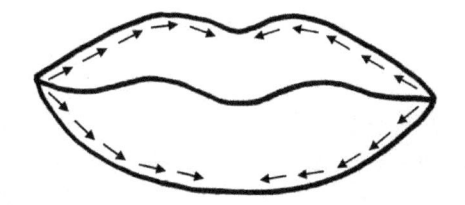

LIP LINER APPLICATION

The application of lip liner is the process of applying pencil to the edge line of the lips. This is done in order to give the lips more definition, or sometimes as a corrective method for irregular shaped lips. When used on the lip line, it can give a sharp and clean edge while giving the appearance of the lips more enhancements. Lining the lips isn't always required unless a defined look, or correction is desired. Using these various techniques when applying lip color in combination with lip liner will give a completed finishing touch.

As with lip color, the health of the lips are important. When lips are in better health they will be smoother, and the liner will provide more definition. When the lips require exfoliation or moisturizing, it's more common to have skips or breaks within the liner application.

Prior to each application the pencil should be sharpened and sprayed using 99% alcohol to kill any bacteria. Keeping a sharp and sanitized lip pencil is also important. It's not recommended to use the pencil with multiple people without first taking the steps of sharpening and sanitizing first. The sharp point will be helpful when creating fine and hard edges.

When the lip pencil is used, it's often easier to control by resting the pinky finger on your mode's chin when applying. This will provide a steadier hand motion during the process.

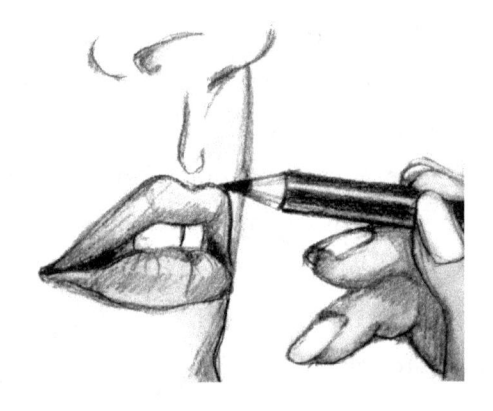

UPPER LIP

The model's mouth should be relaxed. Starting in the center, give the Cupid's bow definition.

Bring the pencil up until you reach the peaks, then trace along the lip line. Take caution not to exceed the edges.

Then trace out, meeting the outer corners of the

model's mouth.

LOWER LIP

From the outer corner, draw towards the lips center.

Repeat from opposite side of mouth.

LIP LINER WITH LIP COLOR APPLICATION

Practicing both the lip liner, and lip coloring applications, they can be used in combination with each other for a great finishing touch to a make-up application.

By choosing to use a liner that is similar to the color of the lips will provide a more defined and consistent appearance. Using a liner a shade darker will provide definition with depth. It's important to remember while using this technique, you want to pull the liner into the lips with a brush in order to give the appearance of depth at the lip line. It will also create natural looking soft edge.

There are colorless and clear lip liners that will help give a soft or natural appearance. The clear liner is usually used with a color since it's clear to help prevent color bleeding, especially popular among mature women.

Keep in mind that additional cheek color may be needed once the lip color has been added. Using a mirror, decide objectively if it is needed or not.

MAKE UP

Using the lip coloring and lining techniques as the last process in the make-up progress, the lips add the finishing touches. In order to stay organized and save time, you should lay out any products required before starting. Sharpen and sanitize your pencil using 99% alcohol, which will provide fine and sharp edges.

As stated in the previous lesson, you want to apply the liner to the natural lip line without exceeding the lips edge. Keeping the pencil sharp is important to get a fine line.

Now follow the point-to-point method and fill in lips with the color of choice.

Then using various combinations of liner and color as described earlier to get different effects.

Using a mirror, view your model. Being able to see them when finished helps you view work form multiple perspectives.

MAKE UP

LIP CORRECTION

Lip correction requires being able to identify, and correct lips with irregularities in shape or size. The main objective is to make the lip balanced, both with it's self and the model's face. There is various shaped lips, it is essential to have knowledge and identify them quickly. Some shapes will be mildly irregular, while others are more noticeable and caused form several irregularities.

No matter the shape, the overall goal is to give the lip a naturally balanced look by correcting the irregularities. The majority of the time only a small adjustment is needed, however, there are situations where more may be required. By reviewing the various lip shapes within this lesson, you will understand the various techniques used to balance the lips and how to apply them.

When correcting an irregular lip shape, extending the lip line past the labial roll may be required. The labial roll is the natural section around the lip that provides natural highlights and dimensions Due to this natural highlight, it's important to pay attention to the labial roll, if it loses it's highlight, then the lips dimension will also be lost. This will cause the lip to appear flat or unnatural.

In the case the labial roll's natural highlight is lost, it will need to be corrected to keep the natural appearance of the lip. This is possible by using a light shade of base

MAKE UP

color, or adding highlight around the new lip line by blending it into a soft edge.

Being able to correct the shape of a lip is extremely important as it helps with balancing the faces proportions, and being able to use a lip pencil will be very helpful with achieving this goal.

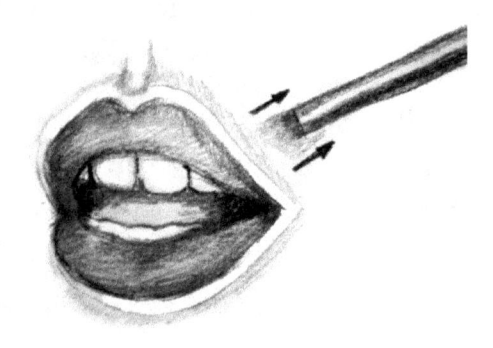

MAKE UP

LIP SHAPES

In the illustration below, many various shapes and appearances that a make-up artist will often come across are shown. It's possible to see a combination of multiple shapes as well. Maintaining the balance of the lips is very important when correcting lip shape.

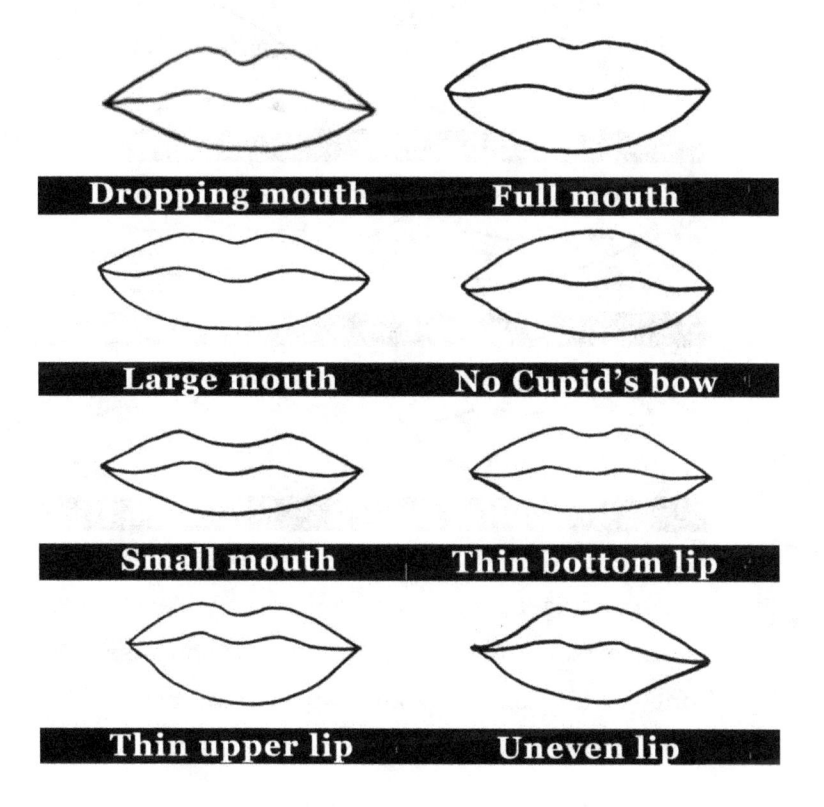

Dropping mouth	Full mouth
Large mouth	No Cupid's bow
Small mouth	Thin bottom lip
Thin upper lip	Uneven lip

In the illustration here, the dotted lines show the location lip liner should be placed in order to reshape or correct the lips shape. Usually the adjustments required are minor, but produce great results.

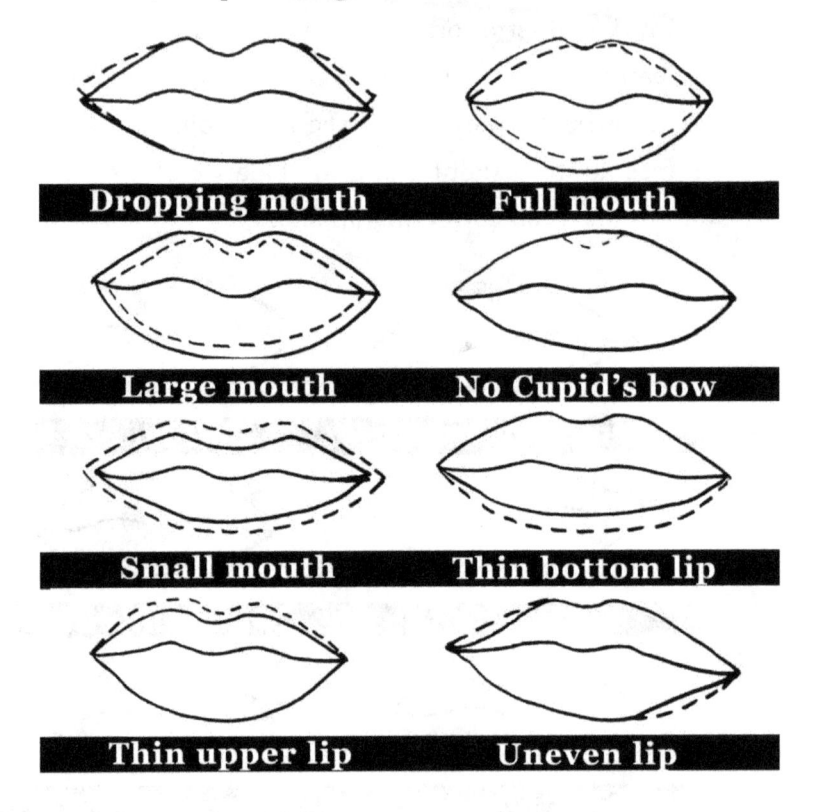

Dropping mouth | **Full mouth**

Large mouth | **No Cupid's bow**

Small mouth | **Thin bottom lip**

Thin upper lip | **Uneven lip**

Correcting lip shapes requires consideration of many characteristics before beginning the process. Stand in front of the model, looking straight at her, ask yourself these questions:

Are her lips well balanced themselves?

Does the upper lip appear larger than the lower lip?

MAKE UP

Does the lower lip appear larger than the upper lip?

Is either side of her mouth drooping?

Does her lips appear thin?

Does her lips appear proportioned with her face?

Is her Cupid's bow defined?

Are the corners of her mouth downward?

Within reason, corrections can be made for most of these situations. Study the following examples. With a sharpened lip pencil, follow the examples, draw in, or outline, to shape and balance the lips, then fill in with lip color, using the point-to-point method as previously described.

After applying, re-check by analyzing the shape of the lips. Look for balance and evenness from side to side and top to bottom. After determining the type of lip shape, use a lip pencil to outline and adjust the shape of the lips as follows.

MAKE UP

EXAMPLE:

If the upper lip is slightly thinner than the lower lip, it is necessary to make the upper lip appear larger by drawing a line where the adjusted lip shape will be. Maintaining the naturalness of the lips is most important. Sometimes, it will take only a slight adjustment to balance both the upper and lower lip.

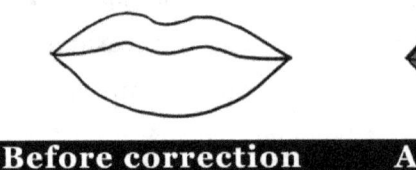

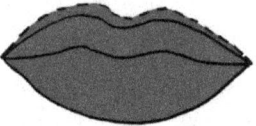

Before correction   After correction

EXAMPLE:

If the lower lip is quite a bit thinner than the upper lip, it is necessary to enlarge the lower lip by drawing and filing it in to balance the lip's top to its bottom.

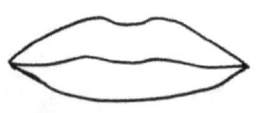

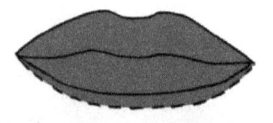

Before correction   After correction

MAKE UP

EXAMPLE:

If one side of the lip is lower than the other, or uneven, it is necessary to draw and fill in the lower side to match the other side. Check the work to be sure that both sides have the same shape.

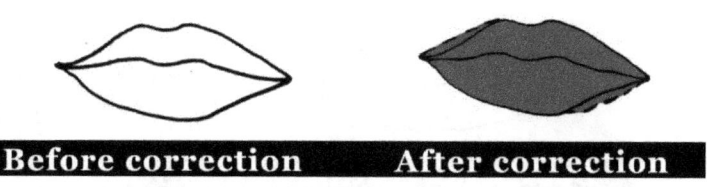

Before correction   **After correction**

EXAMPLE:

If the mouth appears small or out of balance with the rest of the face, it may be necessary to increase the size of both the upper and lower lip. Draw in the adjusted shape and fill in.

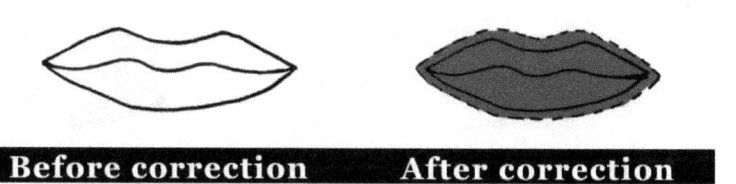

Before correction   **After correction**

MAKE UP

EXAMPLE:

If the mouth appears large or out of balance with the rest of the face, it is necessary to decrease the size of both the upper and lower lip. Draw in the adjusted shape and fill in. The remaining exposed lip will be covered with base.

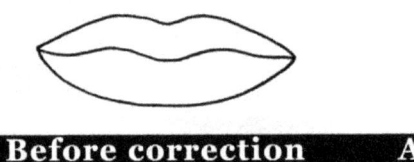

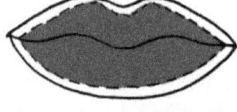

Before correction   **After correction**

Example:

If the upper lip doesn't have a Cupid's bow and is rounded, you will need to create one by drawing it in and creating the Cupid's bow peaks in the center of your lip. Follow it by filling in your lip with color.

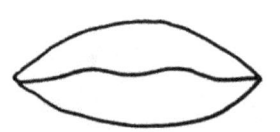

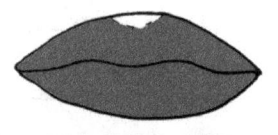

Before correction   **After correction**

MAKE UP

On Color

Light colors will make the lips appear bigger while dark colors will shrink the size of the lip. This is based on the exact theory as shadow and highlights. Shadows push while highlights pull.

In order to blend a darker lip liner into a lighter lip color, simply apply the lip pencil using a dry, clean lip brush to blend the lip liner into a natural lip color. Apply a light lip color to the center of the mouth and simply blend to the lip liner. This will create a soft transition of dark to light and add dimension.

In order to create a fuller look, simply apply a small amount of a light lip color or a shimmery color to the fullest part of the Cupid's bow, and to the center of the bottom lip. If you are wanting a variation of this, simply apply a lighter shade of lip color on the bottom lip.

When it comes to selecting a lip color, the complete look achieved by the artist has to be taken into consideration. An example of this is if a natural look is needed, the color red wouldn't be the correct choice, although a earthy, soft pink would be a good choice.

In order to create a classic look from the fifties period, using soft pinks or peaches wouldn't be the correct selection. A bright red would be the best color to use. As

MAKE UP

with any make-up project, research needs to be done in order to attain accuracy.

Chapter Study Questions

1. Where will you find the Cupid's bow?
2. Lip liner should be applied with what?
3. What is an essential when it comes to apply lip color?
4. What is the natural highlight that surrounds the lips?
5. You can help dry lips by doing what?
6. Where should you start when applying lip liner?
7. What is the actual purpose for applying a lip liner?
8. When you are applying lip color, what position is the brush in?
9. Is lip color in matte texture always?
10. Should lip liner have a hard or soft edge?

MAKE UP

EXAMPLE:

If the mouth has corners that droop, it is necessary to lift them by drawing across the lower lip in an upward motion and slightly filling in the upper lip at the corners, also in an upward motion.

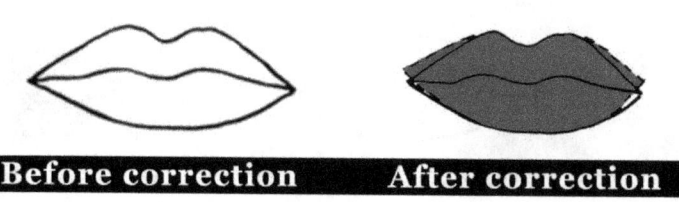

Before correction   After correction

EXAMPLE:

If the lips are full and out of balance with the rest of the face, it will be necessary to decrease the fullness of the lips by drawing inside the lip line on both the upper and lower lip. Once that is done, fill them in with lip color. The remaining exposed lip will be covered with base.

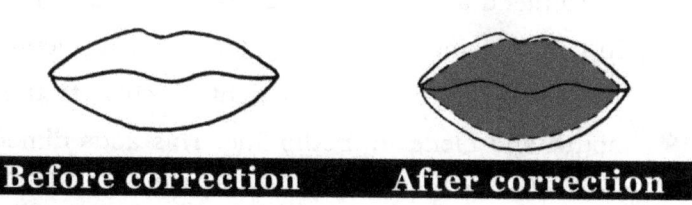

Before correction   After correction

MAKE UP

EXAMPLE:

If the upper lip is rounded and without a Cupid's bow, it will be necessary create one by drawing it in and creating the peaks of the Cupid's bow in the center of the upper lip. Follow by filling in with lip color.

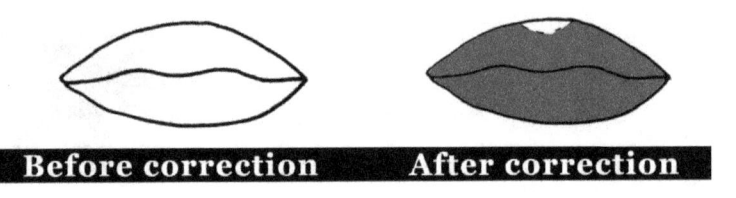

Before correction　　**After correction**

ON COLOR

Light colors tend to make the lips appear larger, while dark colors may seem to diminish the size of a lip; this is based on the same theory as highlights and shadow. Highlights pull, shadows push.

To blend a darker lip liner into a lighter lip color, apply lip pencil using a clean, dry lip brush to blend liner into the natural lip color. Apply light lip color to the center of mouth and blend to the lip line. This adds dimension and creates a soft transition of dark to light.

To achieve a fuller look, apply a dab of a lighter shade of lip color, or a shimmery shade to the fullest part of the Cupid's bow, and to the center of the bottom of the lip. For a variation of this, apply a lighter shade of lip color to the bottom lip only.

When choosing a lip color, the overall look to be achieved by the make-up artist will need to be taken into consideration. For example, for a natural make-up look, the color red would not be the right choice. However, a soft, earthy pink would be a good selection.

To achieve a classic period look of the fifties, soft peaches or pinks would not be the right choice. A bright classic red would be the color to choose. As with any make-up project, research will need to be done for accuracy.

Chapter Study Questions

1. Where is the Cupid's bow located?
2. Lip liner is applied with what?
3. What is essential when applying lip color?
4. What is the natural highlight that surrounds the lip?
5. Dry lips may be helped by what?
6. Where do you start a lip liner application?
7. What is the purpose of applying lip liner?
8. When applying lip color, the brush is in what position?

MAKE UP

9. Is lip color always matte in texture?

10. Should lip liner have a soft or a hard edge?

MAKE UP

CHAPTER 7:
Putting it all together

It is now time to begin combining all the skills and techniques that were developed in the prior chapters for the complete make-up application: a complete look. The make-up artist will begin to develop a consistent pattern for application in order to gain constant results with confidence. The make-up artists will also be able to create glamour, natural, trendy, and fashion looks for both mature and youthful faces.

Straight/Natural Make-Up

Straight or natural make-up doesn't mean that the model isn't wearing any make-up. Natural make-up is soft, clean make-up. The make-up artist will begin putting together some or all of the elements for complete make-up in the following order: foundation/base, powder, eyebrows, eye shadow, eyeliner, mascara, cheek color, and lastly lip color. Select warm or neutral color selections for the cheeks, lips and eyes. Colors should mix well with the model's eyes, hair color, and skin tone. Think more in the terms of beige's, soft peaches, warm browns, light neutral browns, and creams. This isn't the look for heavy eyeliner,

MAKE UP

or glamour eye shadow treatment application. Think more of fresh or clean beauty. The look of the model should enhance the appearance of lips, skin, and eyes without making the model look as if she is wearing excess make-up.

Application

The suggested application for the make-up goes as follows:

- Assess the model's skin and face type
- Cleanse, moisturize and tone the model's face with the right skin care products as needed.
- Assess the model's eyebrows. If it is needed, tweeze, brush, or trim to shape the eyebrows.

Select the right foundation for the model's skin type and the coverage that is desired. Apply the correctly chosen foundation. Use concealer for any skin discolorations if it is needed. Be positive that the foundation is completely blended (for a natural look, the foundation coverage is sheer to medium).

Based on product choice (cream or powder), this may be the right time to set the foundation on the model's skin.

Apply the correct eyebrow color to the brows, defining and balancing the brows.

MAKE UP

Select warm tones to shadow and highlight the eyes, using techniques that are for shadow placement on the eye folds. Use a small amount of product on the eye color applicator, ensuring that the shadows are well blended and soft. The make-up artist will decide to place a drop shadow on the model or not.

Apply the eyeliner using pencil, powder or cake. The application needs to be well blended and light. Apply natural or straight eyeliner with soft edges instead of hard edges, which tend to be more dramatic. Keep the eyeliner shades neutral using a brown or black.

Curl the eyelashes and apply the mascara. Select either the black or brown mascara.

Apply cheek color. Select neutral, warm tones. Keep all the edges well blended to ensure that there are not hard edges on the bottom or top of the cheekbone.

If it is needed, apply lip-liner to bring the lower and upper lip into balance. Use neutral tones that are close to the natural color of the lips.

Apply the appropriate lip color. Select colors that are in similar tones as the cheek color selections. Keep the colors soft and neutral.

When it comes to applying make-up, be aware of the theory that less is more. Basically, only use what you need and do not apply make-up just to apply it.

MAKE UP

Glamour and Fashion Make-Up

The applications of glamour and fashion make-up tend to be more dramatic in the terms of looks. The applications of make-up are used for a dim lighted situation, or for creating a particular character look. Glamour and fashion make-up applications may allow the use of stronger shading and highlights, and vibrant and iridescent color selections, unlike the neutral, muted color selections for a natural look. Although, this doesn't mean that neutral tones can't be utilized. Black is sometimes considered a neutral tone.

Application:

Assess the model's skin and face type

Cleanse, moisturize and tone the model's face with the right skin care products as needed.

Assess the model's eyebrows. If it is needed, tweeze, brush, or trim to shape the eyebrows.

Select the right foundation for the model's skin type and the coverage that is desired. Apply the correctly chosen foundation. Use concealer for any skin discolorations if it is needed. Be sure that the foundation is well blended and that the coverage is sheer to medium,

MAKE UP

based on how the make-up will be shot or viewed.

Apply powder to the model's skin to set the foundation.

Select two to five eye shadow colors to use on the model. Choose what type of shadowing to use on the model; the choices can be clean to smokey, matte to iridescent luster, or soft to intense.

Select an eyeliner and apply it in a position that will enhance the overall look of the make-up. An example of such, for a smokey eye, a choice may be to use fashion eyeliner treatments with a smudged drop shadow that is reinforced with black eyeliner around the eye.

Curl the eyelashes and apply mascara. The make-up artist may want to choose a different color of mascara and may even decide to use false eyelashes.

Apply the cheek color using either gel, cream or powder color.

If it is needed, apply lip-liner to bring the lower and upper lip into balance.

Apply the lip color. If a high-impact look is wanted, apply lip gloss to the top of the lip color.

When the make-up application is completed, examine the look in a mirror; this will give a more visual reading on how the camera may see the make-up.

MAKE UP

The Mature Face

It's important to pay attention to the needs of a mature face when creating a complete look. The mature face shouldn't be heavy or it may look like it was overdone. When it comes to make-up design, less is always more. The look should be flattering to the model, using only natural and neutral colors being from the artist's palette.

It is best to avoid using bright colors because they will look harsh on a mature woman. All the lines should be soft with this application without any hard edges. The final effect of this application should be an enhancement to the mature face, smoothing the skin as well as bringing gentle definition and color to the face.

Application:

Assess the model's skin and face type.

Cleanse, moisturize and tone the model's face with the right skin care products.

Assess the model's eyebrows. If it is needed, tweeze, brush, or trim to shape the eyebrows.

Select the right foundation for the model's skin type and the coverage that is desired. Apply the correctly chosen foundation. Use concealer for any skin discolorations if it is needed. Be positive that the

MAKE UP

foundation is completely blended.

Lightly powder the skin to set the foundation, if needed. The mature face requires very little powder as too much will age the face instead of flattering it.

Apply shadow and highlight to areas that may need to be contoured. Remember, most mature faces will need more highlights than shadows.

Apply cream cheek color. Select a warm tone that looks natural on the model. Use the techniques that were learned in the cheek color chapter for the correct cream cheek color application to the cheekbone.

If needed, add a light dusting of powder to set the make-up. Do not over-powder any area of the face as it may set into creases of the face.

Shape, color and softly define the brows, using either powder or pencil in shades of taupe to warm brown.

Apply the correct eye color treatment to the model, paying attention to the eyes that are recessed and have a heavy fold. Use natural/neutral soft tones to highlight and shade the eyes, like warm apricot in cream, matte finished soft medium browns. Stay away from iridescent colors, as they reflect the light and will draw attention to any part of the skin that may be wrinkled or creepy.

Use wet or dry neutral eye shadows or a cake eyeliner,

MAKE UP

smudge it in order to soften the effect. Pay attention to the eye fold and be sure that the eyeliner doesn't bring notice to the drooping of the eyelid or any heavy folds. The drop shadow should be simple, not heavy or wide. Do not close the corners of the eyes in this application.

Apply a single light coat of mascara in a natural tone to the lower and upper lashes. Avoid any smudges, globs or clumps of mascara on the lashes as well. Comb through the lashes with a lash brush to remove any unwanted or excess mascara, if desired.

Be attentive to the corners of the mouth on a mature face, when applying lip liner. Use corrective techniques for thin lips and drooping corners with needed.

Select a lip liner color in warm tones like coral, rose, apricot, and light berry; the lip liner aids as a barrier to minimize lip color bleeding.

Select a lip color shade. Choose a shade in warm, lighter shades in the similar color families to complement the lip liner and cheek colors used on the model. Matching the lip and cheek colors will help to complement the skin and will look elegant and simple. Use a lip brush to fill in the lip color on the model. Contain the lip color within the border of the lip liner. Matte finishes, gloss, and dark colors are not recommended for a mature model.

Powder the lip to allow the lip color to hold firmly to the

MAKE UP

lips and to minimize bleeding lip color.

After the look is completed, view the model's face in the mirror. Look for any final adjustments that may be needed.

Chapter Study Questions

1. Describe the steps of application for a natural look.
2. Should eyeliner be used in every look?
3. What are trends?
4. Can a glamour eye treatment be used when completing a natural look?
5. Are neutral colors best for natural looks?
6. What eye color treatments are used to create a dramatic look?
7. What type of looks use vibrant colors?
8. When dealing with trendy make-up looks, is it true that it isn't necessary to be concerned with shadow and highlight?
9. Why is it considered important to have a specific order to apply make-up in?
10. Should natural look make-up applications have mostly soft edges?

MAKE UP

CHAPTER 8:
Mature Make-Up

It takes delicate balance and finesse to apply make-up to a mature woman. This chapter will explain the proper techniques and application methods that are necessary to meet the needs of the mature facial structure.

Mature Face Features

As women and men age, their facial structures will significantly change. The main cause for this is gravity, and the pull down effect from gravity. Every aspect of the face is affected by aging, with certain areas being more effected than other areas.

The underneath of the eyes, folds of the eyes, jowls, nasolabial folds, skin of the neck, and corners of the mouth are the most common areas that are effected by the pull down effect; this will create shadows in areas that are unflattering.

The condition of mature skin is another factor. When the aging process begins, the moisture of the skin decreases which will dry the skin out. When the skin has lost moisture, it will also lose the elasticity. Winkles and

MAKE UP

lines will develop. A few of the effects of aging can be improved by a daily regimen of skin care. It is very important for mature skin to replenish its moisture. This will help to keep the skin supple. Age spots and other discoloration of the skin can also be seen on a mature face. A good skin care regimen will enhance make-up application.

There are combined elements that the artist will address when they apply make-up on a mature woman.

Analyzing Mature Faces

The make-up concept for a mature woman is simply to improve the existing features of the mature face. It isn't really to create a youthful appearance, but a great application of make-up can sometimes result in one.

A great artist will develop a critical eye. They will be be able to see details and analyze a mature face to know the negative and positive aspects of a model's face.

The positive aspects will be enhanced while the negative ones are hidden. This will give balance to the mature face while it improves the look of the person overall.

The positive aspects can be excellent skin tone, well-defined brows, long lashes, and bright colorful eyes.

The negative aspects can be heavy folds of the eyes,

bags or puffiness under the eyes, deep set lines across the forehead or nasolabial folds, thinning eyebrows, dark circles under the eyes, deep set lines around the lips, and discoloration of skin tone or age spots. Deep set lines around the mouth is normal for a person who smokes.

When it comes to applying mature make-up, it is truly a matter of seeing and then correcting any negative aspect of the face.

After the artist notices these in the mature face, they will customize the most effective application for the model. This does vary from person to person.

Building the Foundation

Applying a light application of moisturizer before applying foundation will help any dry areas of the skin. Dry skin can prevent smooth application of foundation and can cause it to streak. If too much moisturizer is used, it could cause the foundation to slide on the surface, moving from where it was originally placed.

In most make-up applications, make-up is only applied where it is needed, using the smallest amount possible. This certainly applies when working with a mature face. Since, wrinkles normally exist, applying a heavy amount of foundation will make the wrinkles more noticeable.

MAKE UP

Step 1- Foundation

Analyze the skin and face, apply moisturizer if necessary. Select a foundation color to match. When it comes to a mature face, there could be several skin tone colors. Find a medium shade on the face that is between a darker and lighter shade than is seen. The foundation may need to be mixed in order to get the right match. The undertone is very important. Normally, a mature woman will need some olive in there foundation, as there are some that tend to get an ash tone as they age. In this case, the ash tone can make a person seem unhealthy or cold. Mixing olive in the foundation will help to add a warming tone to the skin.

Place a small amount of foundation on a foundation palette. Load the foundation on a make-up sponge from your palette. Check the sponge in order to ensure an even coverage of foundation. This will help to minimize any streaking during the application.

Start the foundation application on the forehead at the hairline. Work the foundation downwards towards the eyebrows. Add more foundation to your sponge when needed. Cover the remainder of the mature face and neck, while leaving the eye area to be applied last. Blend at the neck to prevent any noticeable changes in color where the make-up stops.

When it is completed, check the application over. Look for any areas that may need to have extra coverage, like age spots that are still showing through the foundation. The areas that you should be aware of are the insides of the corners of the eye and the underneath of the eye.

Step 2 – Camouflage

Using the same techniques that were discussed in the foundation chapter about concealing irregular skin tones, select a color that is close the the skin tone of the model. When working with a mature model it may help the application if the concealer is mixed with a small amount of foundation. This will create a foundation tone relationship and will give more slip to the concealer. Use a palette when mixing.

A small eye shadow or concealer brush will work well when applying concealer to hard to reach areas like the corners of the eyes. This will give the artist more control of the placement of the product.

Once all the areas that needed concealer are covered, use a sponge with foundation, and blend the areas by lightly tapping.

MAKE UP

Step 3- Shadow and Highlight

At this time the face should have even coverage and color. Using either a lighter concealer mixed with foundation or lighter foundation, highlight any deep set lines on the forehead, corners of the eyes, top of the cheekbones, nasolabial folds, corners of the mouth, and temples. Again, this should be a light touch with a little amount of make-up should be adequate enough. Tap these areas with the foundation sponge to blend.

Normally, mature faces will need more highlights than shadows. One area that may need shadow is the the jawline. Combine the shadow color with foundation to make sure that there is the foundation tone relationship.

Mature skin tends to work better with very little to no powder. Powder can actually settle into the face line when it is over used, causing the lines to be very noticeable. Just remember that less is always more.

Eyes

Once the foundation is completed, the artist now has a even, fresh canvas to use for application of all the remaining elements of make-up. Staying with neutral tones for natural looking make-up is the best way to go about mature make-up. Mature women do not work well with bright colors such as greens and blues. They need softness in all forms of make-up, especially when it comes to blending and color.

Eyebrows

The eyebrow shape should be natural and without abrupt arches or harsh edges. To ensure opening the eye, lift and tweeze underneath the brow.

Eye Shadow

The next step after eye framing with the eyebrows is to apply the eye shadow. Notice what type of eye fold the mature person has. It may have drooped with the aging process and should be treated like a heavy fold or a recessed eye. The skin that is in this area may be creepy or wrinkled. It is best to stay away from any iridescent shadow colors. The iridescent colors may show the inconsistencies of wrinkled skin and make the wrinkles more noticeable. The artist is creating an illusion when it comes to most make up; this is certainly the case when it comes to mature make-up.

MAKE UP

Eyeliner

It takes skill to apply eyeliner to a mature eye. A few techniques can give real success. The largest factor is the lack of smooth skin; eye shadow can help to smooth the skin and make it easy to apply the eyeliner.

Mascara and Lashes

Applying a thin layer of mascara is adequate enough to finish the eye make-up.

Eye Applications

Eyebrows

Before adding product, brush the eyebrows in an upwards direction. Tweeze or trim to shape the eyebrow. The color should start at light and build by adding darker shades to keep the dimension. Using a pencil that is combined with eye shadow will help to maintain the softness of the natural eyebrow. Eyebrows are rarely exact, especially where a mature face is concerned.

Eye Shadow

Remember, shadows push and highlights pull. Keep this in mind when searching for any areas that need to be

MAKE UP

pulled forward. This is where the highlight will be placed. Notice the heaviest part of the fold. This is where the shadow will be placed. Use soft yellow or creams for highlight and medium warm browns or taupe's for the shadow. Keep warm tones, avoiding any iridescent colors such as bright blues and greens and black, for a mature application of make-up. These are harsh colors and will make a mature face look hard. Blending all edges in when applying the eye shadow is a must. Be sure to blend the shadow colors to keep the natural and soft look to make-up.

Eyeliner

In order to avoid messy, skipped or hard liner, stay away from the liquid liners. The best for a mature eye is cake liner that is smudged or eye shadows. You can get soft edges with either of those options. Color choices are limited to black, medium browns, charcoal, or dark brown.

When using eye shadow, tap a small wedge or angle brush into the selected eye shadow. Be sure to tap both sides of the brush in order to have an even amount of the product. Follow the guidelines for the eyeliner application, and gently tap the product across the lash line on the upper lid, and follow the contour of the eye.

When using cake liner, use the eyeliner brush. Work

MAKE UP

the dampened eyeliner brush into the product using circular motion, and make a slurry. Follow the guidelines for applying eyeliner and apply it. Soften the edges with a slightly dampened wedge or angle brush to create a soft edge. When dampening the brush, there should not be a lot of moisture on it, this will cause the product to lift back onto the brush and off the eyelid. If there isn't enough moisture, it will cause the product to flake.

Mascara and Lashes

If needed, curl the lashes. The best color of choice for a mature face is either black or dark brown mascara. Do not use bright colored mascara. Apply by following the guidelines that were stated previously. Keep a light application and be sure to apply to both the upper and lower lashes. If using a cream mascara, watch for clumping and keep a consistent application.

Cheeks

Keep the blush/cheek color light on application. Skin that has too much make-up on will have an opposite effect of what you are trying to do, especially on skin that isn't as smooth as it once was.

Soft colors like light apricot or pale rose will add glow to the cheek. Dark colors will have more of a contour effect on a mature woman. Apply a light coat to the cheek with

MAKE UP

blush or a cheek color brush. Start at the hairline and in small circular motions work towards the front of the cheekbone. Follow the guidelines for cheek color application. Be careful to not bring the color too far forward.

Warm colors on make-up applications will bring it to life, where using cool colors will age a person.

Lips

Pay particular attention to the lips. The corners of the mature mouth may show signs of drooping. There may also be lines around the mouth as well that range from slight to quite deep, especially if the person happens to be a smoker. This means that when the lip color is applied it should fill those lines. This is called bleeding. Dark colors will show more bleeding than a lighter lip color.

The lips are the last step in applying mature make-up. After it is completed, analyze and observe the entire application and make any final adjustments.

Lip Color Application

If lines around the lips are noticeable, to minimize bleeding you can apply foundation and powder. Another way that works is to apply lip pencil to the lip lines. This

MAKE UP

acts as a dam to aid in stopping the color from bleeding.

Use a lip pencil that is the same shade as the color that will be used on the lips. Using any corrective methods that have been discussed in the lip chapter. Line the lips and remember to keep the lip pencil sharp. Select a color that is in a matte finish and not glossy. Apply the lip color up to the lip line. Using a soft peach or natural rose color is a great choice. Keep within the lip line and do not go over it. When the lip color is kept within the lip line, a barrier will be created.

This useful method will involve tissue, brush, and colorless powder.

Separate the tissue. Normally tissue is two-ply but for this application you will only need one-ply. Place the tissue on the lips. Using a blush or cheek color brush, apply the powder over the tissue using a tapping motion. This will give a light dusting of powder on the lip color. Using a clean brush, dust off any excess powder and reapply the lip color.

You can repeat this step for long wear lip color.

MAKE UP

Chapter Study Questions

1. How much powder is used on a mature make-up look?

2. What types of colors are good selections for this type of look?

3. Is mature lip color likely to end up bleeding?

4. Do bright or dark colors work with this make-up look?

5. Why is the care of skin important?

6. What type of folds tend to be found on a mature face?

7. How do you deal with age spots?

8. Should you correct the nasolabial fold?

9. Why is uplifting an important effect in mature make-up application?

10. What is the recommended type of eyeliner application?

CHAPTER 9:
Bridal Make-up

One of the most controversial make-up styles happens to be bridal make-up. What is bridal make-up? Basically, it is what the bride wants it to be. A wedding style can be considered a photo shoot or society make-up style. Many weddings are now being video taped and there are even more that are using both to capture their special day. Today there are more themed weddings than there ever has been before, so bridal make-up can be considered character make-up. The make-up that's applied is individualized and it will have to be adjusted for every bride.

The Process

Consultation

There are several things that should be considered when doing bridal make-up and for this reason communication with the bride is the most important part. A consultation with the bride is always recommended to learn what type of make-up look she has in mind.

Use this consultation to gather as much information

MAKE UP

about the wedding as possible, such as:

- The season; winter, fall, summer, or spring
- The time of day; evening, morning, or afternoon
- Location of the wedding(city/state)
- Is it outdoors(ocean, park) or indoors(place of worship, dining hall)
- Colors of the wedding(bridesmaid dresses, flowers, etc.)
- How the hair would be worn.
- If there are hair decorations such as a veil, hat, or flowers.
- Style of the dress; sexy, casual, or formal.
- Color of the wedding dress; warm or cool, white, cream or off-white
- How many people will have make-up application? Is the groom wanting or needing a make-up application?

The bridal consultation needs to consider and include all details of the style of the wedding, so that the make-up is harmonized and not battling with the overall look of the wedding. A normal American bride would have natural soft make-up, that uses soft cool or warm colors, whatever is best with her coloring and possibly the dress. If the bride comes from a different type of culture, discover what would change. An instance of such is a Persian bride, they tend to want darker lips and exotic eyes. When you have a consultation with the bride, find out what she would like.

Do a Make-up Test

A make-up test is always recommended in order to establish a relationship with the bride and to create the make-up design before the wedding day. Once the bride and artist are pleased with the test, it is always good to record the work. Snap a photo of the make-up design, preferably using a Polaroid camera. Take plenty of notes for a future reference.

A make-up test is a great way to be able to discuss the fess; there aren't any set rules – the artist can charge per hour, per day, or by person, whatever you prefer.

It is a wise idea to collect at least a portion of your fees upfront at the make-up test, up to 50%. Include any fees for mileage, travel, parking fees, etc. It is always recommended to collect the full amount of your fees before the wedding, since there tends to be a lot of confusion and excitement during the wedding, and you may have to remind them that you need to be paid, if you are able to find them.

MAKE UP

The Make-up

If this is a springtime wedding, the make-up will normally be in natural, soft shades with soft, glowing cheeks. This helps to create a healthy look, that reminds people of spring. If the wedding is a more formal occasion and is in the evening, the make-up can be dramatic using smoky eyes, or red to darker lips, instead of the natural, clean daytime look that is made with peaches and soft pinks. A period wedding will require make up that fits that time period; a 1940's themed wedding will have natural, soft eyes with thin, long lashes and red lips. Be aware that different cultures will and may impact the style of the make-up. Whatever the choice may be, consider using water-resistant products such as lip stains, foundations, waterproof mascara, lip ink, and maybe waterproof eyeliner more as a safeguard since crying is normal at a wedding.

If the artist does not plan to stay for any touch-ups, then leave a touch-up kit that they can purchase for the bride that includes lip liner, powder, and lipstick. You may want them to purchase this before the wedding.

CHAPTER 10: Airbrush

The simple concepts of operating an airbrush in the application of beauty make-up can give the artist an understanding of the breakdown and mechanical workings of an airbrush. The simple concepts that you are fixing to learn, and with some practice, you can become an artist with a proficient skill with an airbrush.

Airbrush Basics

Many airbrushes were designed to allow water-based enamels, paints, acrylics, make-up, and adhesives to flow easily through them. Any free flowing type of material that has a milk consistency can be sprayed through an airbrush.

Before explaining how to use an airbrush, you should first know how the tool actually works. The airbrush is a small metal tool that is attached to a hose that is connected to a source of air like a compressor. A small trigger or button on the airbrush will allow the airbrush to release air from the tool. The air then moves past the small opening in the tip of the tool and creates a vacuum and then draws the make-up into the stream of air. The make-up and air are then pushed from the tool towards whatever you are painting.

There are two types of airbrushes that will be discussed, they are the single action and the double action airbrush. Many airbrush manufacturers create both styles and even a few more than that. The term single action simply refers to the trigger motion of the airbrush. A trigger has one function only and when it is pressed down, both air and make-up are released from the tool. There normally is a screw or knob on the tool that will allow you to set the amount that is sprayed when you press the trigger. Double action also refers to the trigger motion. When the trigger is pressed down the air is released and when you pull back on the trigger it allows the paint to mix with the air and spray from the airbrush.

There are some airbrushes that come with interchangeable parts and if you want to adjust the spray pattern and the viscosity of the fluid. Thick fluids will need more pressure and a larger nozzle. The pattern size can be determined by the size of the tip or nozzle on the airbrush and the distance that the tool is held from the surface.

Single action airbrushes are very durable and will allow you to spray almost anything through them. What is better is that they are easy to clean an easy to use. The double action airbrush is considered the workhorse in this

MAKE UP

industry and happens to be used by a huge number of artists due to the versatility. It has been used for applying full body paint to painting animatronic skin. Although it is more difficult to use because of the hand-eye coordination.

Be sure to keep your airbrush in good working order and clean. Follow the instructions from the manufacture and it will become a very important tool in your make-up kit.

Air Supply

In order for an airbrush to work, it must have air pushed through it. There are a number of ways to provide air to your tool. The most common way is through a compressor but the real challenge is finding the right one that works for you.

The first option is the compressor motor. These tend to be inexpensive although do not supply an even airflow and can be very noisy.

The next is a compressor with a tank attached to it. This type has an even airflow and motor that shuts off once the tank is filled. The motor of the compressor will only restart in order to refill the tank, although it can be quite noisy while it is filling.

Another option is a silent compressor that has a tank

and a motor. The motor is insulated and tends to be very quiet. Although, this type of compressor is very pricey and it costs around 4 times more than a standard compressor.

The last option is carbon dioxide gas. Although, carbon dioxide isn't really air, art stores will have carbon dioxide in cans about the size of spray paint. You may even purchase carbon dioxide canisters from welding supply stores and these tend to last longer and can be refilled. The canisters come in various sizes from 10 lb, 20 lb, and sometimes larger. The 10 lb tank will last around 10 hours of moderate spraying while the 20 lb will last 20 hours.

Maintenance

Before you place your airbrush down, even if it is a short time, empty the color out of it and run water through it or the right type of solvent depending on what you are using. There may be times when the product will dry inside of the airbrush and then begin to clog it. The airbrushes performance will be affected severely if it isn't cleaned. To completely clean the airbrush, you will need to dismantle it. Refer to the diagrams of each airbrush in order to properly assemble or disassemble it. When the airbrush is taken apart completely, you will be able to clean every part of it.

MAKE UP

Operating the Airbrush

There are three movements that a beginner needs to know in order to become familiar with it. Hold the airbrush so that the tip of your forefinger is resting on the button that will activate the airflow. Press the button down to start the air flow into the brush. For the double action airbrush, pull back on the button to start the airflow. Now you simply move your hand up and down and left and right.

The distance from your work surface and the tip will determine the size of the spray pattern. The further you are from your surface, the wider the pattern; the closer you are to your surface, the thinner the pattern. Build the color gradually, if you add too much product or if the surface is too wet, the product will run.

Airbrush Exercises

Here are some simple exercises that is recommended to try in order for you to gain basic control of your airbrush. The following exercises are created to be done on paper and then the skin and should be carried out as so.

Exercise 1

This has been designed to give you some basic control

over your airbrush. First we will begin the process of making dots. This will help you to gain control. Start on a piece a paper before you begin to move on to skin and use water-based make-up for simple clean up. In order to become familiar with the functions and feel of your airbrush, practice by spraying air from your tool. Now hold your airbrush about an inch from your paper, begin to spray air and slowly pull back on your trigger to begin to introduce the make-up to the paper. Keep practicing this until you are able to place dots accurately without spraying a lot of make-up on the paper. If you pull back too far on the trigger, make-up will pool in one spot causing a puddle. Next try to adjust the size of the dots that you are making as well as the intensity. In order to do this, you will have to allow more make-up to pass through the airbrush and you will have to increase your distance away from the surface. Once you have mastered this skill you will be able to place the color anywhere needed and in any quantity that you need it.

Exercise 2

This exercise will allow you to apply make-up evenly with your airbrush, and be able to blend one color to another. When you are using an airbrush to apply make-up, sometimes you may be applying foundation to an actor's face, or creating an even skin tone over someones body. You will start this practice on paper before you try it on skin. White paper will be able to show the areas where you will need more coverage. Practice by moving the airbrush right and left over your paper. Be sure that you are moving your hand right to left before releasing the color. Otherwise, where you start and stop your movement will cause the coverage to be heavier than in the middle, which will create spots at the beginning and end of your movements. Another way to achieve the same type of result is to work in a circular motion with your airbrush to create a smooth and even coverage over a large area. The final result should be a even and thin application of color without any puddles.

Exercise 3

The final exercise is meant to enable you to be able to apply color in layers. Start by spraying a thin application of color in a horizontal line and about 2 inches in height. Next you will spray another horizontal line with the same thickness but about 1 inch in height and you will overlap the previous line by covering the bottom half of the first line. Lastly, create a third line, with the same thickness but only a half an inch. The result should be a very nice graduation of color from a light on the top to a dark color on the bottom.

MAKE UP

Repeating this exercises over and over again on paper before on skin will give you the confidence and the skills that are needed to use the airbrush in a beauty make-up environment. This is just the start of your efforts to use an airbrush professionally. The airbrush can be used to apply full body make-up or beauty make-up. For beauty make-up use your airbrush when applying the foundation, the cheekbone shadow, the jawline shadow, the cheek color to the top of the cheekbone, and when applying the highlights under the eye.

Chapter Study Questions

1. What is the best consistency for the flowing liquid through an airbrush?
2. Are airbrushes single or double action?
3. The size of a nozzle or tip determines what?
4. Describe a good technique of creating even and smooth coverage over a large area?
5. When would you use an airbrush in doing a make-up application?
6. What is needed to provide air to the airbrush?
7. Why is it important to clean your airbrush after every use?
8. What will vary the size of the spray pattern?

MAKE UP

9. Too much product on a surface will do what?

10. Will an airbrush create only a fine line?

What to Look For In An Eye Cream

Whether you are wanting to deal with wrinkles, dark circles, puffiness, or crow's feet there are plenty of products to help. The best serums and creams will boast special increments that will target your trouble areas. Here is what you should look for:

Aloe Vera

The greatest sunburn treatment around is also known to sooth even the most inflamed, driest skin. When you are wanting to calm, nourish, and hydrate your skin, look for products that list aloe as an ingredient.

Antioxidants

Vitamins A, E, and C, grape seed extract and green tea extract have been proven to neutralize free radicals such as the highly charged oxygen molecules caused by stress, smoking, and by the sun which can cause loss of collagen, dark spots, wrinkles and inflammation. Antioxidants will counteract the free radical damage and boost the cell repair, stimulate collagen production and fade blotches and discoloration.

Caffeine

Drink too much caffeine and you will dehydrate your skin, but when it is used in an eye cream, it becomes a great beauty enhancer. Caffeine has been proven to help reduce puffiness, minimize dark circles and tighten the skin.

Green Tea Extract

Studies have been shown that one of the most effective antioxidants that will neutralize free radicals is green tea extract. It also happens to be a strong anti-aging ingredient.

Hyaluronic Acid

This is a great ingredient that is used for thirsty eyes. Hyaluronic acid works to help plump up the skin and boost skin cells with extra moisture.

Peptide

Peptide increases the elastin and collagen production that helps to keep wrinkles from happening. They are very gentle which makes it a great choice if you have sensitive skin.

Vitamin C

This nifty vitamin has been proven to increase collagen and elastin production and it is a very strong tool against wrinkles. Look for formulas that state that they use ascorbic acid and contain vitamin E in order to boost the effectiveness.

Vitamin E

This strong antioxidant protects, moisturizes, and repairs. Vitamin E is also has calming and soothing properties.

A Word about Retinol

Retinol is a potent Vitamin A derivative and is considered on of the best ways to treat sunspots, fine lines, and wrinkles. Retinol stimulates the cell turnover and will increase collagen production. Although, it can only be used at night due to the fact that it poorly interacts with sunlight. If you have sensitive skin, you should avoid using anything that contains Retinol as it can trigger rashes and redness.

MAKE UP

Natural Eye Treatments

Sometimes some of the best eye treatments are the easiest. When it comes to puffiness or bloating in your face, nothing beats drinking a few cups of cranberry or lemon infused water and avoiding salty meals. You can even find some of the greatest eye beauty boosters from nature just by looking in your fridge or getting into your pantry. Here are a few:

Cold Tea Bags

Had a rough night? Tea bags will certainly help. Steep in hot water for about 5 minutes and then wring them out and place them in the fridge to cool. Lie back with your head elevated and place the cold tea bags on your eyes. The caffeine that is in black or green tea will help take care of the swelling while chamomile will soothe the irritation and redness.

Cucumbers

It is certainly true, sliced cold cucumbers that are placed on the eyes are great for reducing the irritation and puffiness due to their cool temperatures and great astringent properties.

MAKE UP

Jojoba oil

Applied with a cotton ball, jojoba oil is hydrating and a great way to naturally remove make-up. It will easily remove your eye shadow, eye liner and will make a great moisturizer if your in a pinch.

Sleeping with your head elevated

A pillow that will support your neck and head that is elevated will help to promote lymphatic drainage, making sure that fluid doesn't settle in the skin around the eyes. While sleeping flat on your back is good for your back, it isn't so great for puffiness.

Take it off

Because your eye area is really delicate, you should only use a remover that is designed for your eyes to remove your make-up. I would recommend using gentle formulas that include soothing ingredients like rosewater extract and aloe vera. If you are the type to wear long-wear or waterproof make-up, you will need to find a product that is formulated to remove long-lasting make-up.

The best way to apply eye make-up remover is with a cotton pad or ball. A cotton swab can help remove any traces that are left.

MAKE UP

The Doctor says:

There are a lot of amazing products that are out there for your eyes. Although, it can be really hard to find out all your options. I asked Dr. Rosemary Ingleton, a dermatologist, for advice on helping those who have the three most common complaints about beauty.

Dark Circles

Look for eye creams that contain Vitamin K to battle the dark circles under your eyes.

Puffiness

Look for products with green tea extract, Matrixly (an anti-aging ingredient), caffeine, and chamomile are the best out there.

Wrinkles

Search for products that contain alpha hydroxy, hyaluronic acid, Matrixl, neuropeptides, growth factor, and retinol.

Ask a Developer

How long do I keep eye make-up?

MAKE UP

We asked the VP of Global Product Development at Bobbi Brown Cosmetics, Gabrielle Nevin, how long you should wait before you update your favorite product. This is what she shared:

- Powder Eye shadow and Face powder: 2 Years
- Eyeliner: 2 Years
- Mascara: 6 Months
- Concealer and Corrector: 2 Years
- Eye Creams: 6 Months
- Brushes: More then 10 years if properly cared for (Page 15 for instructions)

If in the event of an eye infection, there may be a chance that you need to toss any make-up that has come in contact with the infection. It is always best to consult your doctor.

Basic Eye Techniques

From how to rid yourself of dark circles with corrector and concealer to making your eyes pop with the right liner, here are the foolproof tips to getting amazing eyes.

Corrector

I always get asked, what is one type of make-up that I couldn't live without? My answer is always concealer and corrector. These are the products that can improve your look dramatically. When you apply concealer and corrector, you will appear less tired, instantly brighter and refreshed. This is why I call them the secret of the universe. Combining both products will make them the rock stars of make-up.

If you happen to have chronic dark circles or simply had a super late night, adding a layer of corrector under the concealer. Corrector is pink or peach based under eye make-up that was created to brighten, counteract, and neutralize discoloration around the eye.

Choosing the Right Shade of Corrector

Bisque or pink colored correctors work well with women who have pale to medium skin tones. Women who have warmer skin tones should look for a peach colored corrector. Dark peach or dark bisque corrector works great on darker skin tones. If your corrector appears to be too white after you have applied it, it isn't the right shade and you should go darker. If it happens to be too yellow or it doesn't instantly brighten your eyes, go lighter.

Applying Corrector

Begin with applying a small amount of a fast absorbing

MAKE UP

eye cream and then apply your corrector with a brush to the inner corner of your eye area, applying it on where you see the darkness. Then gently blend with your fingers and then clean your brush with a tissue before you apply your concealer. Corrector and concealer do not work if they get mixed together. They should be layered.

Corrector and Concealer Tips

Always use a small amount of a quick absorbing hydrating eye cream before you apply the corrector and concealer. Be sure that the cream isn't too greasy and is fully absorbed or your make-up may slide off.

Your skin tone will vary from summer to winter. If you change to a slightly darker foundation in summertime, you may need to have a slightly darker concealer also.

Layer and pat your concealer with your fingers to help blend it into your skin. Never pull or tug at the delicate skin around your eyes. Dab and Softly blend.

A white or pale yellow sheer powder on top of your concealer will set it in place.

Concealers

Yellow based concealers will work magic when it is

applied over your corrector with a clean brush. They will lighten the dark areas, cover up any redness, and make you look completely rested instantly. They will give you an immediate lift by simply brightening your eye area.

Choosing your Shade of Concealer

In order to select the right shade of concealer, look for a yellow based creamy formula that is just one shade lighter than your natural skin tone. Women who have various skin tones tend to benefit from a yellow based formula. The yellow tends to blend well into the skin and makes you look awake without you looking like you are wearing a ton of make-up.

Applying Concealer

Using a clean brush, apply your concealer on the top of your corrector, making sure that you get as close as you can to the eyelashes and in the socket and inner corner of the eyes. Blend with your fingers until it appears smooth.

Finish with Powder

Set the concealer with a powder in order to keep it from creasing and to make it last longer. Simply apply a light dusting of a yellow toned powder over your concealer with an eye sweep brush. If you are very pale, try to use a translucent powder. Go with a peach based powder if you have a darker skin tone.

Troubleshooting

After applying the corrector and concealer and if it still looks dry under your eyes, you didn't start out with enough eye cream. If anything smears then you most likely applied too much eye cream and should add more powder in order to finish.

Skincare

It helps to understand skin when you are a make-up artist, since it will be the canvas that you work on. If you prepare and look after the skin, then the make-up that you apply will sit better and will last a lot longer. It's fully recommended to study the skin at the level of a beautician, this will help you to understand make-up application a lot better.

It isn't really necessary to carry a skincare range for every skin type in your make-up kit. Although, it is important to be able to control and manage each skin type to the advantage you need. Many make-up artists and tutors at AOFM are huge fans of Dermaloica. It is a brand

MAKE UP

that knows the importance of skin and makes products that make the artists' job a lot easier as well as offering ongoing training for artists that are lucky enough to get included on their artist list. The following pages will guide you through all the essential skincare products for an artists' go to list.

When you are choosing a skincare range, choose one that isn't heavily perfumed and is okay to use on sensitive skin. Models constantly have make-up applied and removed and sometimes their skin can become sensitive. It is also a good idea to carry a good-quality range if you plan to work with celebrities, which is another reason make-up artists turn to Dermalocia.

When doing videos, beauty and fashion shoots, celebrity make-up, prerecorded television, and bridal make-up, it is best to always use a full range of products that include toner, moisturizer, and cleanser, unless a celebrity requests a preferred brand and products. Shooting on location or live television sometimes requires moisturizer and wipes to save time. Fashion shows, if there is time, will use a full range, but when they are pushed for time, it is always best to carry wipes.

Products and Preparation

It is very important to pay attention to oily and dry

MAKE UP

skin. Dry skin will need moisture and oil put back into it so the skin preparation and products that contain moisture and oil will help to make the make-up last longer. If you don't treat dry skin, there may be flaking which can ruin the foundation. Oily skin needs products that can help reduce oil and shin. Make-up and skincare products containing oil will cause the shine to be very visible and the make-up to slide, thus making the make-up hard to manage.

Cleansers

An ultra calming cream cleanser is a gentle and effective cleanser that is soft enough to be used to remove any eye make-up. It is even convenient when you are on location as it can be removed without the use of water. Face wipes like Simple and MAC can also be used instead of toner and cleanser for speed convenience. These are usually what is on photo shoots and backstage to remove make-up efficiently and quickly.

Toners

Use a convenient spray toner that is moisturizing, refreshing, and gentle. It will help to prepare the skin for a moisturizer and doesn't need to be removed.

MAKE UP

Treatments for Lips and Eyes

Look for a firming vitamin packed type of treatment that contains silicone, which is like a primer, will help to moisturize sensitive skin and smooth wrinkles that are around the lips and eyes. Lucas Pawpaw Ointment is a great thing to use on chapped, dry lips.

Treating the issue (optional)

There are some skins that may require some additional treatment for problem areas. For dry skin or to add moisture, use a hydrating booster before you moisturize. This can also be used on the lips. Sensitive skins requires using a gentle treatment for reducing any redness and calming the skin. If it is mature skin or premature aging, using a firming serum or booster can help to reduce the appearance of annoying fine lines and wrinkles. For skin that is prone to spots and breakouts, using a clearing spot treatment is very effective to help reduce breakouts. Dermalogica has pre-moisturizer boosters for various conditions.

Moisturizers

Select a moisturizer according to your skin type. If you

have chronically dry skin, select a concentrated, rich moisturizer. If you have dry to normal skin, using a medium weight moisturizer like Dermalogica's Skin Smoothing Cream is great to smooth and hydrate your skin. If you have oily skin, you will need a light hydration formula that will reduce the appearance of oil and will help to close the pores.

Tinted Moisturizers

Using a tinged moisturizer is used to provide a sheer cover to help even out the skin tone as well as moisturize the skin. It is great for people who do not like to wear foundation, but would still like a little coverage.

Beauty Serums

Serums are only used as part of a facial treatment. Similar to a moisturizer, a serum is a liquid that is used for treating skin conditions like discoloration, dehydration, fine lines, and redness. They contain highly concentrated ingredients that are then absorbed into your skin deeper and quicker than an intensive effect. The high concentration of the ingredients will penetrate into your skin, providing you with long lasting and dramatic results.

In order to use, simply apply a drop of serum to your

fingertips and gently massage it into your skin in the morning and at night, and then follow up with your normal moisturizer. You do not have to use more than a drop or two to cover your whole neck and face. You will most likely feel an immediate change in your skin the first time that you use a serum. Your skin may feel smoother, softer, and maybe a little tighter.

Exfoliates

Your skin is always generating new skin cells at the bottom layer and are sending them to the surface. As your skin cells rise to the surface, they gradually die and become filled with keratin. The skin cells filled with keratin are important because they will protect our skin during the creation of new skin cells. As we begin to age, the process of cell turnover begins to slow. Cells begin to pile up unevenly on the skin's surface and will give it a rough, dry, dull type of appearance. Exfoliation is beneficial because it removes all the old cells and reveals the younger, fresher skin cells that are below it. It also helps allow expensive facial products such as serums easier to absorb into your skin.

Only use products that are made for the face as some exfoliates are made for your body and can be irritating and too abrasive for your face. A fine powder exfoliant that will

MAKE UP

become a paste when it is mixed with water will smooth the flaky dry skin and remove the dead skin cells. The best method to use is exfoliating gloves or synthetic scrubbing sponge that is made for the face. To do this, simply rub your face gently with the sponge in a circular motion. Avoid scrubbing under your eyes, where the skin is very thin and can be damaged very easily. The residue that is left can be removed with damp cotton wool pads or warm water.

Exfoliating can cause your skin to dry out and dry skin is just an invitation for wrinkles. When you over exfoliate, you are risking bursting delicate blood vessels that are under the skin, if they burst, your skin may always appear flushed.

Face Masks

A face mask can make a huge difference between good and great skin. There is a mask that is appropriate for every skin type. Facial masks will help to exfoliate your skin and remove the build-up of sluggish cells. A face mask, as well as daily skin washes will keep your pores unclogged and will help to remove blemishes by stimulating blood circulation. When the seasons begin to change, your skin will change, so you may need to switch the type of facial mask that you use when the weather changes. Many masks are best when they are applied once or twice a week.

Clay Masks

These masks are best for those who have oily skin because they will draw out the impurities and toxins as well as being essential for keeping the skin clear.

Peel-off Masks

These are intended to gently remove the dead skin cells. Peel-off masks will leave your complexion radiant and refreshed and work with all skin types.

Paraffin Masks

These are for softening and hydrating the skin. The paraffin wax masks are good for all skin types and help blood circulation which will brighten your complexion.

Pore Strips

These are usually used for the instant removal of blackheads, dirt, and oil. If you want to minimize your pores, you should use pore strips. They have double the effectiveness of a pore cleansing face wash and are handy to have in your kit to prevent breakouts and clogged pores. You can get instant results and the pore strips can be used up to three times a week.

Applying a Mask

Try to use a facial mask about three times a month. Applying a mask will require a specific technique, but many of us have no clue about that, we just put it on our faces. The first step is to use a spatula or a flat wide brush. Avoid using your hands!

Start by applying your mask with a spatula or brush from the center of your face and work outward using even strokes. Be careful to avoid your lips and the sensitive area around your eyes.

Leave the mask on for about 20 minutes, unless there is a certain time frame that is stated on the packaging. Never leave the mask on for more time than is recommended by the manufacturer. There are some ingredients in it that could harm your skin if they stay on longer than they are needed.

To remove your mask, moisten with a little bit of water and gently rub off the skin. Work on one area at a time. If you are using a peel-off mask, you simply peel it off. Finish by rinsing your face with plenty of water using circular motions to remove any left behind residue.

MAKE UP

Primers

A primer is a product that is used to prepare your skin before foundation is applied. They are all silicon based for the most part. The silicon in the primer is used to fill in fine lines and pores, to create a smooth base for applying all the other make-up. The main benefit from using a primer is that it will help the make-up last longer on the skin.

There are various types of primers that are available, just like there are different types of moisturizers for the various skin types. Primers tend to work best on cleansed prepared skin and if the skin happens to be very dry, a primer can be placed on the skin after the moisturizer.

Types of primers can include mattifying for oily skin to help control the shine, hydrating to help moisturize the dry skin, and simple primers to help plump the skin to give it a youthful look. Many primers will contain SPF and they can come in a various textures like mousse, gels, lotions as well as mineral powder for those who have sensitive skin.

The professional make-up artists including those who happen to be in the fashion industry, will tend to have a large range of primers in their kits for use on various jobs. Even though the fashion industry will look for models who

MAKE UP

have plump and young skin, they are prepared to do touch ups in between the shots. There are some occasions where the primer will be needed, such as shooting in an outdoor editorial and that is where primer with SPF comes handy. Models who have dehydrated or are tired, we see this a lot when it comes to fashion week, may need hydrating primer in order to smooth and soothe the skin.

Primers are popular in the film and television industry and they tend to range with ages of actors and presenters are used. Also while being on the set or on location and under warm lights for long time periods will require make-up to last longer in between the normal touch ups.

With the increasing industry of high definition film and television the make-up that is used by presenters and actors will need to be more natural, but effective. As powder tends to look heavy when on television or film, an artist can use a mattifying primer to help prevent shine and reduce the unnecessary excess powder and continuous touch ups. Also, more mature presenters and actors will need a silicon based primer like Prep + Prime Skin produced by MAC, will help to smooth over the fine lines to form a smooth canvas for foundation to go on the skin flawlessly. The Becca Line and Pore Corrector is an oil free, skin tone that can help to help minimize the lines and pores around the nose and eyes for a smooth foundation application.

MAKE UP

Foundation & Concealer

Foundation

The main focus for using foundation is to even the skin tone and skin color. How an artist wants the skin to appear varies from face to face – the appearance will differ. On one project an artist may want the skin to have a nice healthy glow while on the next an old fashioned matte, full coverage type of foundation or the following one may need to have a natural look, as if the model is not wearing make up at all.

Selecting the product that you need to use is considered one of the bigger challenges that a new make-up artists can actually face. Here is a small guide to help sort out their confusion.

Full Coverage

This is the type of foundation that will give the skin an appearance of being flawless. A good full coverage can effectively cover discoloration, blemishes, and cover scars almost like a concealer, over the entire face. The foundations will also work on black or Asian skin tones.

In order create flawless foundation on any skin, simply dilute the stick foundation or full coverage by combining with a sheer tinted moisturizer.

Applying Sheer Coverage

Sheer foundation will allow skin to look unmade and natural. It will even out the skin tone, but will allow freckles, beauty marks, and more to be seen, allowing the effect of having a make-up free face.

Oil Control/ Oil Free

This type of foundation is perfect for people who happen to have oily skin as the formula can help to eliminate shine by giving the skin a matte finish. Usually when something says oil free it simply means that it doesn't contains any mineral oils or lanolin, these are the oils that have a tendency to cause sensitivity and clog pores.

Illumination

This is the type of foundation that will give a luminous and glow type finish on the face. Some of the illuminating foundations can contain tiny glitter or pearl particles. When working on photo shoots it may cause the skin to have a greasy appearance.

MAKE UP

Moisturizing

The best foundation for normal to dry skin types, it will give the hydration and will work on those who have mature type of skin.

Cream to Powder

This type of formula has a more traditional texture, although it will usually come in a compact. It will applied as a creamy texture and will dry to a powder type finish. Cream to powder formulas will give a medium finish which tends to be ideal for those skin types that seem to need more coverage than the typical liquid foundation but just not as much as a full coverage.

Powder Based

This type of foundation is great on oily skin since it has no moisture or liquid in it, this type will give a non-reflective matte appearance to the skin. Another type of advantage to this is that is able to be used with a brush in order to set the make-up.

Mousse

This whipped product will give a light coverage as well as a matte finish or natural glow and when applied to the skin, it has a very light, airy feel.

Tinted Moisturizer

This is a combination of some color and moisturizer. This is great for an evening out type of skin tone. It will give a light coverage and will absorb into your skin easily.

Try to use tinted moisturizers if you have a dewy complexion, and you happen to be looking for a sheer light wash in order to even out the blemishes.

Concealers

This is used to cover imperfections and blemishes. Once it has been applied, the concealers will cover a heavier coverage than normal foundations and will help to cover dark circles under the eyes. When you are selecting a concealer, you should consider the color and consistency. It should be lightweight and creamy as well. The product will need to glide on smoothly and shouldn't require excessive rubbing. Find the correct shade and blend it that it looks flawless and not obvious. It should be able to match your skin tone exactly. Concealers look most natural when it is worked in sheer layers and built up gradually.

If you happen to be covering under the eye circles that

MAKE UP

are major, you are going to want a formula that will provide a heavier coverage. If you happen to have sensitive skin then you will be able to select a formula that will contain only a pure mineral pigment colors with no dyes, starch, talc, and oils.

Applying Foundation

Before you apply foundation, be sure that the skin has been just been cleansed and then moisturized. After you have applied the moisturizer, wait just a few minutes for it to be absorbed into your skin before you begin the application of foundation. If your face is sticky and damp, it may cause your foundation to look uneven and clogged up. Try to use a non-sticky type of lotion that isn't greasy or use a good facial oil like Bio Oil.

Dab small dots of foundation on your face around the forehead, on the cheeks, your chin, and down the nose.

To minimize pores, always apply the foundation using downward strokes. Sweep over your ears and under your jaw and don't cover up any of your natural rosy cheeks or freckles.

Use a sponge, your fingertips, or a brush to blend the foundation. Be sure that it is well blended enough that it will create a flawless, natural look. Be sure to always apply the foundation lightly and quickly. Even and smooth

MAKE UP

strokes will help to prevent the colors from having a clogged look.

Check the application in a natural light in order to be sure that your foundation is well blended. If you believe that you need to have more coverage, then simply apply a concealer in the certain areas instead of using more foundation.

Concealing Dark Circles

Use a yellow tinted concealer to hide dark purple circles and tan or mauve concealers to hide brownish circles. The tan and mauve are the best for blending into black or dark skin. There are even light blue and green concealers that will hide red under the eye circles.

Apply multiple dots of concealer under the eyes and then tap and press in using your finger, but never rub. Apply the concealer on the other uneven spots of your face, including the chin and around the mouth and nose if needed and then tap in.

Be sure to pay close attention to the area where the eye meets the bridge of the nose. This is the area that tends to have the darkest circles and will need more concealer.

Apply your foundation that you wear in order to even out the complexion of your skin. Blend it as you normally

MAKE UP

would, without paying any attention to the underneath of your eyes. Once the foundation is in place, you will be able to see if there are any dark circles that are still visible. Tap in a heavier coverage as in step one if they are still visible.

Powder any concealed area with a translucent powder, using enough so that the concealer doesn't look shiny or sticky. Using a soft brush will help with the application.

If you are wanting better coverage and more staying power, let your concealer set for 5 to 10 seconds after you apply it and before you begin blending.

Mix a highlighter with your concealer to add in brightness under the eye or use a brightening concealer. This will camouflage just like your concealer, while adding wonderful highlights to your face.